100 Questions & Answers About Leukemia

Edward D. Ball, MD
Gregory A. Lelek

JONES AND BARTLETT PUBLISHERS

Sudbury, Massachusetts

BOSTON   TORONTO   LONDON   SINGAPORE

World Headquarters
Jones and Bartlett
Publishers
40 Tall Pine Drive
Sudbury, MA 01776
info@jbpub.com
www.jbpub.com

Jones and Bartlett
Publishers Canada
2406 Nikanna Road
Mississauga, ON L5C
2W6
CANADA

Jones and Bartlett
Publishers International
Barb House, Barb Mews
London W6 7PA
UK

Library of Congress Cataloging-in-Publication Data
Ball, Edward D. (Edward David), 1950–
    100 questions & answers about leukemia / Edward D. Ball, Gregory A.
Lelek.
        p. cm.
Includes index.
    ISBN 0-7637-2038-0
    1. Leukemia--Popular works.   2. Leukemia--Miscellanea.   I. Title: One
hundred questions and answers about leukemia.   II. Lelek, Gregory A. III.
Title.
    RC643.B355 2002
    362.1'9699419--dc21

                                                2002009864

The authors, editor, and publisher have made every effort to provide accurate information.
However, they are not responsible for errors, omissions, or for any outcomes related to the use
of the contents of this book and take no responsibility for the use of the products described.
Treatments and side effects described in this book may not be applicable to all patients; like-
wise, some patients may require a dose or experience a side effect that is not described herein.
The reader should confer with his or her own physician regarding specific treatments and side
effects. Drugs and medical devices are discussed that may have limited availability or be controlled by the Food and Drug Administration (FDA) for use only in a research study or clinical
trial. The drug information presented has been derived from reference sources, recently pub-
lished data and pharmaceutical research data. Research, clinical practice, and government regulations often change the accepted standard in this field. When consideration is being given to
use of any drug in the clinical setting, the health care provider or reader is responsible for
determining FDA status of the drug, reading the package insert, reviewing prescribing information for the most up-to-date recommendations on dose, precautions, and contraindications,
and determining the appropriate usage for the product. This is especially important in the case
of drugs that are new or seldom used.

Acquisitions Editor: Christopher Davis
Production Editor: Elizabeth Platt
Cover Design: Philip Regan
Manufacturing Buyer: Therese Bräuer
Composition: Northeast Compositors, Inc.
Printing and Binding: Malloy Lithographing
Cover Printer: Malloy Lithographing

Printed in the United States of America
06 05 04 03 02   10 9 8 7 6 5 4 3 2 1

Contents

When physicians and scientists discuss the outcome of their work for a lay audience, they tend to be uncomfortable. The complexity of the vocabulary in which they conduct their day-to-day work makes ordinary communication difficult for scientists. There is, in addition, a feeling in the scientific community that the public has a sense of frustrated expectation that the pace of biologic discovery has not led to more breakthroughs, and this sense of frustrated expectation leads to difficulty in accurately presenting the true advances that have been made.

100 Questions & Answers About Leukemia by Edward Ball, MD and Gregory Lelek therefore fills an important need in improving the ongoing dialogue between the scientific community and the lay public. The complex vocabulary that has been developed over the past 50 years to deal with the remarkable advances in medical research and, in particular, with the dramatic advances that have occurred in the diagnosis and management of the leukemias, have made understanding these advances difficult for the non-medical public. The question-and-answer format of this book makes the centrally important information about leukemia, its diagnosis, and its treatment extremely accessible. The lucid style adopted by Dr. Ball and Mr. Lelek, and the clarity of their presentation, demystify the complexities of the molecular information that is required for a general understanding of this group of diseases.

The demystification of the language of leukemia provided by this remarkable book brings to mind the revelations that occurred with the deciphering of the Rosetta Stone early in the 19th century. The Rosetta Stone, which was discovered in the Nile Delta in 1799 during the Napoleonic invasion of Egypt, contains a long inscription in three languages: Greek, Aramaic, and Egyptian hieroglyphics. At that point in time the skill to read and understand Egyptian hieroglyphics had been lost. For over 1500 years, no one understood what meaning hieroglyphic symbols contained. Following discovery of the Rosetta Stone, it was studied for over 23 years by the French linguist, Jean François Compillion, in an attempt to understand the language of Egyptian hieroglyphics. Eventually, Compillion was able to establish the hieroglyphic symbols for the name of the Egyptian king Ptolemy V, which was present in the Greek and Aramaic parts of the inscription. He then tested this 7 letter hieroglyphic word against another name, Cleopatra, and now had 13 hieroglyphic symbols. Later came the deciphering of the name Alexander, and soon all of Egyptian hieroglyphics were accessible to readers everywhere.

The comprehensive approach of Dr. Ball and Mr. Lelek to an understanding of what for many people is the hieroglyphic symbolic language of science and medicine has the impact of a modern-day Rosetta Stone. The text is finely tuned, the vocabulary is direct and useful, the vivacity of the underlying research is preserved, but without the burden of being perceived as an impenetrable abstraction.

It is important to recall while reading this book that the remarkable advances in the treatment of leukemia we now enjoy have occurred over the brief span of the past 50 years, beginning with the pioneering work of Dr. Sidney Farber in Boston. In the period between 1947 and 1949 the first successes in the treatment of leukemia occurred, accomplished by a team headed by Dr. Farber. We are now on the verge of curing many forms of leukemia, particularly leukemia in children. This book summarizes the advances we have made, and the step-wise progress that has been made to bring us the great improvements that have occurred since 1947.

But even with these remarkable advances, we are not anywhere close to where we want to be. Charles Dickens might describe our time as the Season of Light, and the Season of Darkness; the Spring of Hope, and the Winter of Despair. The reality is that every eighteen-and-a-half minutes, someone somewhere in the

United States still dies from leukemia. And that someone is a man or a woman, a boy or a girl, a husband or a wife, a father, a mother, a son, a daughter, a grandchild. Or that someone is surely a friend of you, the reader of this book. It is the sheer weight of this harsh statistic that brings us together in reading this book, as we ponder the wealth of information provided to us by Dr. Ball and Mr. Lelek.

Ronald McCaffrey, MD
Lecturer in Medicine
Harvard Medical School
and
Lowell General Hospital
Lowell, Massachusetts

Hearing the words, "I am sorry, you have leukemia" in 1997 was the start of the ride of my life. A new way of existence began. A strange (medical) language had to be conquered, making it possible to communicate with those who were treating me. I had to develop completely unknown characteristics for me—patience and trust. Worse, I had to rely on others for survival, a terrible thought at age 45—not to mention dealing with pain, depression, and many months on chemotherapy drugs.

I am here, and I am alive. A wonder to those around me. To get to this point, significant challenges were overcome, not just by me, but by others around me who gave so much of themselves to let me continue to live. No appreciative words can be said that would generate the feelings that I have for all the help and love I was awarded. I am grateful to my fantastic support partners at work, the medical staff from Fred Hutchinson in Seattle and UCSD in San Diego, the continuous prayers from my church members, my donor, and most of all my wife—the greatest caregiver and best friend anyone could have.

Why must we face such challenges? Surely we can do without all this trouble and grief. God apparently thinks not. Romans 5:3,4 says, "…we also rejoice in our sufferings, because we know that suffering produces perseverance; perseverance, character; and character, hope." When we run into problems and trials, we discover that they are good for us—they help us learn to be patient. And patience develops strength of character in us and helps us trust God more each time we use it, until finally our hope and faith are strong and steady.

Finding "the" treatment or regimen that will work against leukemia is the constant challenge for physicians and support staff—a challenge made all the greater by the fact that we are all unique creations, and thus what works for one may not for others. Fine-tuning treatments, learning from experience, and envisioning new ways of healing are the "art" portion of medical arts and sciences. Although we understand some of the ways that the entire body, mind, and spirit interact in disease and health, there are still many aspects of disease and healing that we don't yet grasp—and there are many great advances that still lie ahead, to be uncovered in the future by the diligent searching—and occasional inspirations—of the people who seek cures for leukemia and other cancers. In the end, though, it is the Master, the One who created us all, who is the true doctor and healer.

Gregory A. Lelek
May 2002

We wrote *100 Questions & Answers About Leukemia* in the hope that readers like you would find this book useful in understanding leukemia and its many treatments. As we hope we have made clear, leukemia is not just one disease; it is a family of diseases. The seriousness of a diagnosis of leukemia depends in part on the type of leukemia in question. A diagnosis of acute leukemia usually implies that immediate treatment is necessary. This can be very difficult for a patient and the family, as there is little time to learn about the disease before embarking on therapy. On the other hand, a diagnosis of chronic leukemia is often an incidental finding that can be confusing because the patient may have few symptoms, if any.

We have tried to encompass the multitude of questions that a patient and the family will have for a diverse set of situations, and we hope that the information provided in this book will supplement the information provided by the patient's doctor. Perhaps this book will stimulate you to think of additional questions—that's something we want to encourage, as a well-informed patient can better care for himself or herself. At the same time, this book is not meant to take the place of your doctor's advice; it is very important that you trust in your physician, and we encourage you to seek information from your healthcare provider(s) as a primary source. There are many controversial issues in the treatment of leukemia, so it is important to understand what your doctor's philosophy is regarding the treatment of your particular disease.

Researchers around the world are working hard to understand the basic biology of leukemia in order to develop better treatments. For instance, the recently approved drug Gleevec™ is an outstanding example of what can be achieved once the basic mechanism of a disease is understood. We are all hopeful that similar advances will be made in the other types of leukemia. We encourage you to contact your elected officials to voice support for continued and enhanced levels of funding for basic research into the causes or treatment of cancers and leukemia.

Ted Ball, MD
Gregory Lelek

PART ONE

The Basics

What is leukemia?

What is blood composed of, and what blood cells are affected by leukemia?

How does leukemia affect my immune system?

More ...

1. What is leukemia?

Leukemia literally means an excess of white blood cells in the blood. Leukemia is a malignant disease (that is, a cancer) of white blood cells in which there are too many white blood cells in the blood and the bone marrow. There are several types of leukemia, but they all have in common the uncontrolled growth of one of the several types of white blood cells. There are four major subtypes of leukemia and several rare forms. The major kinds of leukemia are:

1. Acute myeloid leukemia (AML)
2. Chronic myeloid leukemia (CML)
3. Acute lymphoblastic leukemia (ALL)
4. Chronic lymphocytic leukemia (CLL)

Other, rare types of leukemia include hairy cell leukemia, Sezary cell leukemia, plasma cell leukemia, prolymphocytic leukemia, and the leukemic phase of lymphoma.

Leukemia is a serious and life-threatening disease. It might seem odd that having *too many* white blood cells is dangerous because white blood cells fight disease. So how can you have too much of a good thing? As described later, cancerous white blood cells do not behave the way normal white blood cells do, so they cannot fight disease effectively. If the bone marrow (see Question 5) overproduces these cancerous cells at the expense of normal cells, the leukemia patient may soon end up with insufficient numbers of the normal cells to fight off daily infections. Furthermore, the overproduction of these abnormal white blood cells leads to decreased production of other important blood cells, including red blood cells and platelets. For this reason, leukemia is a very serious, potentially fatal condition.

2. What is blood composed of, and what blood cells are affected by leukemia?

As you know, blood is a red liquid that is vital to life. Blood is composed of water as well as a multitude of different proteins, including antibodies and important hormones and transport molecules; nutritional products, such as sugars, fats, and amino acids; and most importantly for the topic of this book, living cells. The major types of blood cells are **leukocytes** (also known as **white blood cells**), **red blood cells** (cells that contain hemoglobin and carry oxygen to the tissues), and **platelets** (cells necessary for blood clotting and formed in the blood marrow) (see Figure 1). All blood cells are manufactured in the bone marrow, growing from a cell

Leukocyte

A white blood cell or corpuscle.

White blood cells

A blood cell that does not contain hemoglobin; also called leukocyte.

Red blood cells

Hemoglobin-containing cells that carry oxygen to the tissues.

Platelet

A cell formed by the bone marrow and circulating in the blood that is necessary for blood clotting.

The Basics

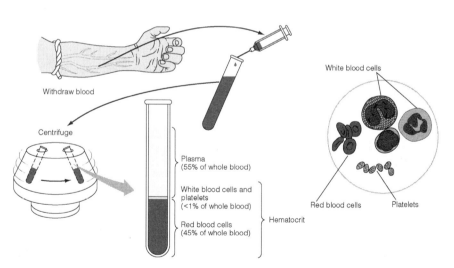

Figure 1   Blood composition. Blood removed from a person can be centrifuged to separate plasma from the cellular component. Red blood cells constitute about 45% of the blood volume, except at higher altitudes where they make up about 50% of the volume to compensate for the lower oxygen levels. Reprinted from Chiras DD, *Human Biology: Health, Homeostasis, and the Environment* (Fourth Ed.). Copyright © 2002, Jones and Bartlett Publishers, Inc.

Lymphocyte

One type of white cell; lymphocytes are weakly mobile cells made in lymphoid tissue.

T lymphocytes

Lymphocytes that directly attach themselves to virally infected or transformed cells to cause their destruction.

Antigen

Substance capable of stimulating an immune response.

Monocyte

A type of white blood cell that is transported to tissues, where it turns into a macrophage.

Macrophage

A cell derived from a monocyte that functions to protect against infection and noxious substances.

Microorganism

An organism of minute, microscopic size.

Antibody

Any of the body's immunoglobulins that are produced in response to specific antigens.

known as the hematopoietic stem cell (see Question 32). Leukemia is a malignancy (cancer) of the white blood cell. However, there are several types of white blood cells (Figure 2).

Lymphocytes are one type of white blood cell that can be further broken down into **B lymphocytes** and **T lymphocytes.** B lymphocytes, which are the minority, make antibody molecules, which are secreted by these cells and can then attach to substances called **antigens.** An antigen can either be a soluble molecule (a protein dissolved in liquid blood) or possibly a protein attached to or part of a foreign cell such as a bacterium, fungus, or cancer cell (a cell the divides and reproduces abnormally with uncontrolled growth). T lymphocytes directly attach themselves to cells infected or transformed by viruses to help destroy them.

Another type of white blood cell is the **monocyte,** or, once it is specialized (differentiated) in tissues, the **macrophage.**

The monocyte is important for a couple of reasons. The first is that monocytes are highly effective at digesting foreign antigens, such as those from an invading virus, and presenting them to T lymphocytes to generate an immune response in order to protect the individual. This is the primary way that long-term immunity against invading microorganisms works. The second function of monocytes is that they are able to ingest, or engulf, invading **microorganisms** (organisms of minute, microscopic size) or cells that have been targeted by **antibodies.**

TABLE 7-2

Summary of Blood Cells

Name	Light Micrograph	Description	Concentration (Number of Cells/mm³)	Life Span	Function
Red blood cells (RBCs)		Biconcave disk; no nucleus	4–6 million	120 days	Transports oxygen and carbon dioxide
White blood cells Neutrophil		Approximately twice the size of RBCs; multi-lobed nucleus; clear-staining cytoplasm	3000 to 7000	6 hours to a few days	Phagocytizes bacteria
Eosinophil		Approximately same size as neutrophil; large pink-staining granules; bilobed nucleus	100 to 400	8–12 days	Phagocytizes antigen-antibody complex; attacks parasites
Basophil		Slightly smaller than neutrophil; contains large, purple cytoplasmic granules; bilobed nucleus	20 to 50	Few hours to a few days	Releases histamine during inflammation
Monocyte		Larger than neutrophil; cytoplasm grayish-blue; no cytoplasmic granules; U- or kidney-shaped nucleus	100 to 700	Lasts many months	Phagocytizes bacteria, dead cells, and cellular debris
Lymphocyte		Slightly smaller than neutrophil; large, relatively round nucleus that fills the cell	1500 to 3000	Can persist many years	Involved in immune protection, either attacking cells directly or producing antibodies
Platelets		Fragments of megakaryocytes; appear as small dark-staining granules	250,000	5–10 days	Play several key roles in blood clotting

Figure 2.   Summary of blood cells. Reprinted from Chiras DD, *Human Biology: Health, Homeostasis, and the Environment* (Fourth Ed.). Copyright © 2002, Jones and Bartlett Publishers, Inc.

The third type of white blood cell is the **granulocyte**, a term that refers to the large numbers of granules in these cells. The most common granulocyte is a cell called the **neutrophil**. The neutrophil is highly effective at recognizing and killing bacteria and other microorganisms. The absence of neutrophils is perhaps the worst consequence of acute leukemia because your body's ability to fight off bacterial and fungal conditions is virtually nonexistent when the body is empty of neutrophils.

Granulocyte

White blood cell with a large number of granules.

Neutrophil

The most common granulocyte, a type of white blood cell.

The Basics

All blood cells arise from a class of cells called stem cells (see Question 32). The bone marrow stem cell is called the hematopoietic stem cell, referring to its ability to make all the cellular elements of the blood. The stem cell is capable of renewing itself during cell division, but it is also capable of undergoing a process called **differentiation**. At the start of this process, the stem cell goes through several stages of development, which result in more specialized stem cells with limited differentiation capabilities, which finally give rise to each of the various blood elements. Leukemia appears to be initiated by **genetic** events (i.e., inherited patterns for certain characteristics) occurring in the stem cell at a particular stage in development. Thus, the type of leukemia that arises has something to do with the exact nature of the genetic event and the cell in which the event occurs. If the malignant transformation occurs in a neutrophil precursor, the disease **acute myeloid leukemia** (AML) arises. If the disease is begun by a particular molecular event in the stem cell, a disease known as **chronic myeloid leukemia** (CML) develops. If the disease is initiated in a stem cell that has differentiated into the lymphoid lineage, the resulting leukemia will be a lymphocytic leukemia of either B cells or T cells, known as **acute lymphocytic leukemia** (ALL). Finally, a particular subset of lymphocytes appears to be susceptible to malignancy giving rise to the disease **chronic lymphocytic leukemia** (CLL).

Differentiation

The process where the stem cell goes through several stages of development.

Genetic

Refers to the inherited pattern located in genes for certain characteristics.

Acute myeloid leukemia

Rapidly growing leukemia affecting mature white cells.

Chronic myeloid leukemia

A slow-growing leukemia of mature white blood cells, associated with the Philadelphia chromosome.

Acute lymphocytic leukemia

Rapidly growing leukemia affecting mature lymphocytes.

Chronic lymphocytic leukemia

A slow-growing leukemia that affects mature lymphocytes.

3. How does leukemia affect my immune system?

Leukemia depresses your **immune system** (a complex system by which the body protects itself from outside invaders that are harmful to it) somewhat indirectly. On one hand, the presence of the large numbers of leukemia cells crowds out the normal cells of the immune system, which causes **immunosuppression** (i.e., lowered resistance to disease). In addition, the treatment of leukemia may further depress the number of normal immune system cells and further contribute to immunosuppression. In general, the immunosuppression is specific for fairly common microorganisms, such as bacteria and fungi that are all around us naturally. When the levels of normal white blood cells that ordinarily keep us from getting infected are decreased, these common bugs can become quite aggressive and can enter the blood and tissues.

4. What are risk factors for leukemia?

Leukemia seems to arise from damage or alterations occurring in the DNA that, in turn, affect various genes. Thus, DNA-damaging agents are known initiators of leukemia. These include certain chemicals, such as benzene and other solvents; ionizing radiation; and some other organic compounds, including, paradoxically, chemotherapy drugs themselves, that is, drugs used to treat other cancers. In fact, so-called **secondary leukemia** (i.e., that caused by chemotherapy) is fairly common in patients previously treated with certain types of chemotherapy for breast cancer, Hodgkin's disease, and multiple myeloma. The incidence of secondary AML approaches 5% in certain

Immune system

Complex system by which the body protects itself from outside invaders that are harmful to it.

Immuno-suppression

Condition of having a lowered resistance to disease. May be a temporary result of lowered white blood cells from chemotherapy administration.

Secondary leukemia

A malignancy that occurs in patients previously treated with certain types of chemotherapy.

subgroups of patients treated in this manner. Obviously, this is a great tragedy, and efforts to modify chemotherapy regimens to reduce the incidence of secondary leukemia are ongoing. Leukemia is also age dependent. Children are at higher risk for ALL, and adults are more at risk for CLL. Adults are increasingly at risk for AML as they age; the incidence of this disease increases even more rapidly in patients over the age of 60 years. CML begins to occur in young adults to middle-aged adults, but is slightly less common in older adults. Certain **congenital diseases** are associated with a higher incidence of leukemia, including Down syndrome, Bloom syndrome, and ataxia telangiectasia. Leukemia also occurs in twice as many patients who smoke cigarettes compared with those who do not.

Do electrical power lines cause leukemia? This issue has been raised numerous times in the past. Many studies have been conducted, but none has found any evidence to support the theory that living near power lines can cause leukemia. There are occasional reports of "clusters" of cases of leukemia in a community. These sorts of events raise the question of whether some local exposure to toxins or poisons, radioactivity, or electrical power lines is the culprit. However, studies are usually inconclusive, and often, no good explanation for the clustering is ever discovered.

In fact, in most patients with leukemia, the disease does not have any identifiable cause. That is, most patients have not worked in occupations that exposed them to toxic substances, they have not taken known leukemia-inciting drugs, and they have not been exposed to radiation above the usual levels that an

Congenital disease

A disease existing at or dating from birth.

In most patients with leukemia, the disease does not have any identifiable cause.

average person would be exposed to in the course of life, such as from dental x-ray studies or an occasional chest x-ray study. It seems that an accident occurs during cell division in the bone marrow in which a mutation occurs in the genome that suddenly triggers the onset of the disease. Perhaps it is related to the extraordinarily high rate of cell division that takes place every day in the bone marrow and the blood, leading to the inevitability that occasionally accidents will occur during the process of duplicating the DNA during cell division.

5. What is bone marrow?

Bone marrow is a soft, fatty substance inside bones where all of the blood cells are made. Some of the bone marrow is so-called red bone marrow, which is where the blood cells are made. Some is so-called yellow bone marrow, which is largely replaced by fat. The red bone marrow is predominantly found in the skull, vertebral bodies, ribs, sternum, and pelvis. There is a complicated architecture inside the bone, where the bone marrow cells reside. Although the bone marrow cavity is separated from the blood circulation by a membrane, they are still in direct contact with each other. As blood cells are made in the bone marrow cavity, they gradually acquire the ability to mobilize from the marrow into the blood, which is percolating through the bone. Thus, the bone marrow is the site of blood cell production. All blood cells, including lymphocytes, originate from a stem cell (see Question 32) that resides in the bone marrow.

Bone marrow
The soft, fatty substance filling the cavities of the bones. Blood cells are made here.

PART TWO

Facts About Leukemia: Risks, Diagnosis, and Effects

Are there different types of leukemia? Why is one called acute and one called chronic?

More ...

6. Are there different types of leukemia? Why is one called acute and one called chronic?

The four major types of leukemia are acute lymphocytic leukemia (ALL), acute myeloid leukemia (AML), chronic lymphocytic leukemia (CLL), and chronic myeloid leukemia (CML). The term **acute** is applied to leukemias that present abruptly and are characterized by large numbers of very immature, undifferentiated cells that, if untreated, rapidly lead to death of the patient. The term **chronic** applies to leukemias that grow more slowly and less dramatically, thus leading to a much longer life span for the afflicted individual, even without treatment.

Acute Lymphoblastic Leukemia

ALL is a cancer of lymphocytes that often begins in a rapid, dramatic manner. ALL is the most common cancer in children, but it also occurs in adults. There are three different subtypes of ALL, based on the appearance of the leukemic or blast (imperfectly developing) cells. These subtypes are termed L1 (most common in children), L2 (most common in adults) and L3, the most aggressive, also called Burkitt's-Like Leukemia. The treatment of ALL is complicated. Multiple chemotherapeutic drugs are used in a phase called **induction chemotherapy** to induce a **remission** (a complete or partial disappearance of the signs and symptoms of the cancer) (see Table 2 and Questions 23 and 24). After this, **intensification chemotherapy** using more chemotherapy drugs is required to achieve the desired goal of a cure. This phase of therapy is designed to eliminate any leukemia cells that were

Acute

Occurring suddenly in a short period of time.

Chronic

Occurring more slowly and less dramatically than acute conditions.

Induction chemotherapy

The initial phase of treatment using medication.

Remission

Complete or partial disappearance of the signs and symptoms of disease in response to treatment; the period during which a disease is under control.

Intensification chemotherapy

Use of additional cancer drugs after remission to eliminate any remaining cancer cells.

missed by induction chemotherapy. In addition, the spinal fluid often is invaded by ALL cells, leading to the need to either treat or prevent spinal fluid involvement with ALL, using drugs introduced into the spinal fluid through a lumbar puncture or through a device inserted into the brain called an "Ommaya reservoir." After a remission is achieved, patients with ALL must continue to undergo treatment for a full 2 years.

The cure rate of *childhood* ALL is very high, approaching 75% of patients. The cure rate in *adult* ALL patients is not quite as good, but it has improved steadily over the years. One subgroup of patients with ALL has a somewhat worse prognosis: those having the Philadelphia chromosome in the leukemia cells. These patients are usually referred for a **bone marrow transplant**, described in Part 4. In the absence of the Philadelphia chromosome, the cure rate for adult ALL is approximately 40% with chemotherapy alone, and there is increasing evidence that bone marrow transplantation improves the results of chemotherapy in adult patients (see Questions 32–40).

The cure rate of childhood ALL is very high, approaching 75% of patients.

Bone marrow transplant

A procedure in which the bone marrow of a leukemia patient is replaced by another person's marrow.

Acute Myeloid Leukemia

AML usually affects adults. The incidence increases with age, and many patients develop AML as a consequence of treatment for other cancers. This disease has a very rapid onset, with obvious symptoms such as fatigue, fever, infection, and bleeding. Untreated, it is rapidly fatal. However, treatment with chemotherapy is highly effective at achieving complete remission (see Questions 21 and 22). Therapy must be initiated as soon as possible in a hospital setting. **Complete remissions** (total absence of disease) are obtained in 50% to

Complete remission

Total absence of disease.

80% of patients, with older patients having less favorable results than younger patients. There are eight subtypes of AML, as defined by the French American British (FAB) system, labeled M0 through M7. One of the subtypes, M3, is treated with chemotherapy and a differentiating agent called all-*trans*-retinoic acid (ATRA) (see Question 23). The other six subtypes are treated in a fairly consistent manner. Induction chemotherapy (i.e., initial chemotherapy), usually consisting of cytosine arabinoside and one other drug, is used to induce a remission. After remission is achieved, **consolidation** (i.e., repeated cycles of chemotherapy) must be pursued, or almost all patients will **relapse** (i.e., experience a reappearance of cancer after a disease-free period). Consolidation can consist of more chemotherapy, given in "cycles" usually at least twice at approximately monthly intervals. Consolidation may also include **autologous** (using cells from the patient's own body) or **allogeneic** stem cell transplantation (using cells from another's body) (see Questions 35 and 36). The overall cure rate for all patients with AML is only 25%. However, certain subgroups fare much better, depending on the patient's age, the prognostic factors, and the exact treatment that the patient receives.

Chronic Myeloid Leukemia

CML is a disease primarily of adults. It is manifested by a high white blood cell count, and sometimes by a high platelet count. The disease is often diagnosed by chance because it is a chronic, slow-growing process that does not produce any symptoms before the white count starts to rise. CML usually evolves into a more aggressive phase first, called accelerated phase, then a worse phase called **blastic crisis**. Blastic crisis refers to the tendency of CML cells to lose their ability to differentiate into

Consolidation

Additional chemotherapy after remission, often given in cycles.

Relapse

The reappearance of cancer after a disease-free period.

Allogenic

Using another person's cells.

Autologous

Using one's own cells.

Balastic crisis

Inability of immature cells to develop into mature cells.

mature white blood cells. At this phase of the disease, the cells behave very much like cells in AML—they grow rapidly, replacing the normal bone marrow cells, thus leading to low platelets and red blood cells. This phase of CML requires treatment similar to AML, but actually has a worse prognosis than AML. Once the acute phase has occurred, if a remission is achieved with chemotherapy (including the new drug Gleevec, described further below), a bone marrow transplant should be strongly considered at this point.

CML is currently undergoing a revolution in treatment. Previously, patients could be treated with an oral hydroxyurea for a short time to decrease the white blood cell count, and sometimes, they received interferon alpha. Bone marrow transplantation was frequently used in the first, chronic phase of their disease to attempt to cure it, and in fact, transplantation is considered the only known curative therapy for this disease (see Questions 32–42). Recently, the new drug Gleevec (see Question 22) has been approved by the United States **Food and Drug Administration (FDA),** the federal agency responsible for approving and regulating medications, foods, and other products for human consumption. This oral drug, which is relatively free of side effects, produces remission in a high proportion of patients with this disease. It is presently unclear how long this remission will last and whether some patients will develop resistance, which means that the medications that produced remission previously will no longer induce or maintain a response to cancer. As mentioned above, the natural history of CML is that the relative slow progress of the disease gives way to a more acute form of the disease, the blastic phase that is similar to AML. The current question

Food and Drug Administration

A federal institution charged with approving and regulating medications, foods, and other products for human consumption.

with Gleevec is whether it will prevent the onset of blast crisis.

The role of bone marrow transplantation is being re-evaluated at this time because of the use of Gleevec. Patients over the age of 45 to 50 are generally not recommended for transplantation before having a trial of Gleevec. Patients under the age of 45 years with a suitable donor may still wish to consider allogeneic bone marrow transplantation as the known curative therapy, though currently many to most patients are giving Gleevec a chance first. If Gleevec works well, many patients are electing to continue on Gleevec at this time. However, if and when the disease process accelerates, or if resistance to Gleevec develops, allogeneic bone marrow transplant is still the only known curative therapy for CML.

Chronic Lymphocytic Leukemia

CLL is a disease that exclusively affects adults. It is unusual for patients to be diagnosed with CLL under the age of 40, and most patients who are diagnosed are over the age of 60. This is a slowly progressing disease in which the lymphocytes gradually increase in the blood, and eventually in the lymph nodes and spleen. The natural history is a very slow but progressive accumulation of these abnormal yet innocuous lymphocytes. As in other leukemias, the problem arises when the normal blood cells are sufficiently suppressed by the proliferating lymphocytes. Treatment of CLL is also undergoing an evolution because of the introduction of new drugs. Patients are being treated with oral chemotherapy agents, or possibly an intravenous agent called fludarabine (see Questions 23 and 24). Biologic therapy, including monoclonal antibodies and gene therapy, is being introduced in the treatment of CLL (see Question 27). Some patients may undergo bone marrow transplantation, which can be curative in CLL but is limited to relatively young patients with suitably matched donors (see Questions 32–42).

7. What is myelodysplastic syndrome? Is it related to leukemia?

Myelodysplastic syndrome (MDS) is a disease of the bone marrow stem cells in which the normal maturation of blood cells is altered. The cause is unknown, but exposure to chemicals, solvent, and toxins may be responsible for some cases. The syndrome is recognized by the finding of low blood counts; usually two or more of the major blood cell elements are present in low levels in the blood. As the disorder progresses, blood transfusions may become necessary. MDS often leads to acute myeloid leukemia (AML). Roughly one third of MDS patients will eventually have AML. The other two thirds will eventually succumb to complications relating to their low blood counts, such as infection and uncontrolled bleeding.

Treatment of MDS is generally **supportive** (i.e., with the goal of preserving the strength of the patient) because there is no proven treatment that directly treats the underlying disease. **Hematopoietic growth factors,** such as granulocyte colony-stimulating factor (G-CSF, Neupogen; see Question 43) and erythropoietin (Procrit), may help some patients by elevating the blood counts. Drugs such as thalidomide are currently undergoing clinical trials to determine their ability to help patients with MDS (see Question 29). Another

Myelodysplastic syndrome

A disease of the bone marrow stem cells in which the normal maturation of blood cells is altered.

Supportive treatment

Treatment with the goal of preserving the strength of the patient.

Hematopoietic growth factors

Drugs that increase blood cell counts.

experimental treatment involves the use of an anti-serum generated to T lymphocytes, called antithymo-cytc globulin (ATG), which has shown some promise.

At the time of **diagnosis** (the process of identifying a disease by its characteristic signs, symptoms, and laboratory results), a doctor estimates the future course of the disease (i.e., the **prognosis**) and potential for the patient's survival by considering certain features of the disease. These include the percentage of blasts in the bone marrow, the existence of certain cytogenetic abnormalities (see Question 18), and the number of **cytopenias** (low blood counts, either red blood cells, white blood cells, or platelets).

Patients with advanced MDS may be treated as if they have leukemia (because they almost have leukemia anyway). This treatment may restore relatively normal bone marrow function, similar to a remission in leukemia. At this point, autologous bone marrow transplantation may be considered to try to extend the remission (see Question 35). Relatively young patients with an histo-compatibility antigen (HLA)-matched sibling should strongly consider an **allogeneic bone marrow transplantation** (bone marrow transplantation using marrow from another person's body) rather than chemotherapy. This procedure is curative in about 50% of cases.

8. What is a blast?

A **blast** is an immature white blood cell that normally represents an early phase of the normal differentiation process that occurs in the bone marrow. Patients with AML or ALL have excess numbers of these cells in the bone marrow and usually the blood as well. *In fact, it is the presence of large numbers of these cells that allows*

Diagnosis

The process of identifying a disease by its characteristic signs, symptoms, and laboratory findings.

Prognosis

A prediction of the course of the disease; the future prospect for the patient.

Cytopenia

Low blood count.

Allogeneic bone marrow transplantation

Bone marrow transplantation using marrow from another person's body.

Blast

An immature white blood cell that normally represents an early phase of the normal differentiation process that occurs in the bone marrow.

the diagnosis of leukemia. The goal of treatment of the leukemia is to decrease the numbers of these cells to normal levels ("normal" means that fewer than 5% of the bone marrow cells are blasts). Sometimes, it is difficult to tell the difference between normal and malignant blasts when the numbers of blasts are low. More specific tests, such as flow cytometry and cytogenetics (see Question 18), are then used to help distinguish normal from leukemia-related blasts. Your doctor will monitor the levels of blast cells in your blood and bone marrow to assess the status of your leukemia and its response to therapy. It is almost always abnormal to have blasts in the blood. Therefore, your doctor will monitor your blood counts (tests to measure the number of red blood cells, white blood cells, and platelets in blood) and look for any blasts periodically during the treatment of the leukemia and afterward to ensure that the disease is still in remission.

9. What is a platelet?

A **platelet** is a tiny cell that is found in the blood. It is responsible for plugging up small holes that might develop in the blood vessels, and therefore, it is the first defense against bleeding. Platelets originally come from a cell in the bone marrow called a megakaryocyte. Patients with acute leukemia commonly have *low platelet* counts; low platelet counts carry a higher risk for spontaneous bleeding (bleeding with no obvious cause). Therefore, the number of platelets is monitored, and if it is particularly low, platelet transfusions (see Question 50) may be given to keep the platelet level to a suitable level. Patients with CML may actually have high platelet counts when the disease is first diagnosed. Despite this, sometimes the platelets don't work as well

Platelet

Blood cell that stops bleeding and heals injuries.

as they should, so bleeding may occur in CML as well. The platelet count in patients with CLL is normal in the early stages. In later stages, it is often low, either because of decreased production of platelets in the bone marrow or because of increased destruction of platelets from an **autoimmune process** (i.e., when a person's immune system reacts against tissues in his or her own body). This autoimmune process may be treated with **immunosuppressive therapy** (i.e., therapy to decrease the response of the immune system; this treatment is intended to treat the autoimmune process), including prednisone, intravenous immunoglobulin, and splenectomy (removal of the spleen).

Autoimmune process

A reaction of a person's immune system against tissues in his or her own body.

Immunosuppressive therapy

Therapy to decrease the response of the immune system.

10. How common is leukemia?

Fortunately, leukemia is a relatively uncommon form of cancer. Currently, leukemia represents about 3% of all cancer in the United States and has an annual **incidence** (the number of new cases of leukemia occurring during a certain period) of about 31,000. The acute leukemias and the chronic leukemias occur with about the same frequency. However, because patients with CML and CLL on average live longer than those with AML and ALL, the **prevalence** (the number of people alive at any moment) of chronic leukemia is greater.

Incidence

The rate at which a certain event occurs, e.g., the number of new cases of a specific disease occurring during a certain period.

Prevalence

The number of people alive with a particular disease at any moment.

Children are more likely to develop ALL than any other form of cancer in general. AML is the second most common leukemia in children, but is much less common than ALL. Although a rare form of juvenile CML occurs in infants and very young children, CML and CLL do not commonly occur in children.

Young adults are more likely to get AML or CML than ALL or CLL. It is very unusual for someone to contract CLL before the age of 40. However, CLL then becomes increasingly common with advancing age, as do all of the leukemias. In fact, the incidence of AML and ALL increases sharply after the age of 60 years. Therefore, as the population continues to live longer, it is expected that leukemia will be diagnosed more often in the upcoming decades. Table 1 illustrates the expected incidence of each type of leukemia in the year 2002 in the United States, as projected by the American Cancer Society.

Table 1   Expected incidence of leukemia in 2002

Leukemia	Age At Onset*	Incidence
AML	65 years	10,600
CML	50 years	4400
ALL	2–3 years, 65 years	3800
CLL	55 years	7000

*Indicates **median** age, that is, the number at the exact midpoint of the spectrum. Half the cases are below and half are above the median age.

11. Is leukemia inherited? Does it run in families?

The vast majority of patients with leukemia have no family history of leukemia. Furthermore, there is no evidence that leukemia can be passed on to the children of a person with leukemia. That said, there are occasional families with two or more members who have developed leukemia or related illnesses. This phenomenon suggests that there might be a genetic predisposition to develop leukemia, analogous to the known increased susceptibility that some people have to develop certain other forms of cancer, such as breast

The vast majority of patients with leukemia have no family history of leukemia.

cancer. However, at this time, the genetic or molecular basis for leukemia susceptibility is unknown. People with certain genetic diseases such as Down syndrome, Bloom syndrome, and ataxia telangiectasia are more susceptible to leukemia for as yet unknown reasons (see Question 4).

Leukemia occasionally occurs in pregnant women, and most commonly, it is either AML or CML, because the childbearing age coincides with the usual age of onset of these diseases. Obviously, the diagnosis of leukemia in a pregnant woman presents a very serious medical problem and is an emotional tragedy for the parents. What to do regarding therapy depends on when the illness is diagnosed, that is, at what stage of the pregnancy. If the diagnosis is made during the first trimester, termination of the pregnancy may be considered because the woman cannot usually wait over 6 months to begin therapy. Chemotherapeutic drugs are known mutagens and **carcinogens** (substances that initiate or promote the development of cancer). Thus, they should not be used in the early phases of pregnancy. A woman in the second or third trimester may be treated supportively (i.e., to maintain her strength) until childbirth if the disease is not too aggressive. However, if she has AML, she may need to be treated with chemotherapy before delivery. This has been done many times with no clear detriment to the child. On the other hand, waiting to treat until delivery places the mother at greater risk of dying from the leukemia.

Carcinogen

Any substance that initiates or promotes the development of cancer.

12. Is leukemia contagious? Can leukemia be acquired through a blood transfusion?

No. The only exception to this is the rare virus HTLV–1, which can cause a rare form of T-cell disease with some features of leukemia. It is found in certain areas, such as the Caribbean and Japan, and it is transmitted by sexual and bodily fluid contact. However, for the common forms of leukemia, there should be no fear that contact with others could spread the illness.

You may wonder if an animal disease, such as feline leukemia, causes leukemia in humans. Many viruses cause cancer, including leukemia, in animals. However, these viruses have never been found to be present in any humans with leukemia. Again, there is absolutely no evidence of transmission of leukemia to a human being from an animal.

In a **blood transfusion**, the red blood cells are replaced in the bloodstream when a person's own bone marrow is unable to replace them. Because there is no known external cause of leukemia, such as a virus, the only way leukemia could be acquired through a blood transfusion would be by the direct introduction of leukemia cells into the recipient. However, because the cells of a random blood donor would be seen as foreign to the recipient, they would be destroyed immediately. There is simply no evidence that leukemia has ever been acquired from a blood transfusion.

Blood transfusion
Replenishment of red blood cells in the bloodstream when one's own bone marrow is unable to replace them.

13. Does diet play a role in my getting ill?

There is no evidence that any dietary exposure or deficiency can influence the onset of leukemia or its behavior once it is diagnosed. A balanced diet, meaning a diet containing the recommended proportions of the various food groups (vegetables, grains, dairy products, and meat) and vitamins, is certainly recommended for a leukemia patient (as it is for anyone!). This is because a healthy body will help you tolerate

Facts About Leukemia

the treatment you may need for your leukemia. But caution is advised for the use of any special diets in the hopes of improving the likelihood of cure. There is no credible evidence that eating a special diet will "cure" your disease. Dietary supplements should be avoided unless your doctor specifically advises you that it is safe to take them, and the FDA does not regulate or approve of most supplements, allowing unsubstantiated, often erroneous (incorrect) claims to go unchallenged (see Question 54). Of course, if you are "neutropenic," meaning that your body is depleted of important disease-fighting white blood cells, you will be told to avoid fresh fruits and vegetables because they may harbor dangerous microorganisms that could cause illness (see Question 15).

Of course, a discussion of a healthy lifestyle must mention issues such as cigarette smoking, alcohol use, and exercise. Smoking cigarettes will not help you in your fight with leukemia. For one thing, your lungs will be more susceptible to infection. For another, your heart may be affected if it has to work harder to pump blood because of the effects on your lungs. Alcohol use needs to be avoided or restricted to very small quantities, and you should particularyly avoid it when you're in an especially vulnerable condition, such as when you are experiencing low platelets or white blood cells. Alcohol affects the ability of the marrow to regenerate and also depresses the function of normal white blood cells and platelets. If you are already a smoker and find that you suddenly need to be treated for leukemia, nicotine patches can be used to decrease the side effects of sudden smoking cessation.

There is no evidence that any nutritional factor causes leukemia, but cigarette smoking has been found to increase the incidence of AML by twofold. An excellent article summarizing the roles of nutrition and physical activity in cancer prevention can be found at the American Cancer Society's web site at *www.cancer.org*.

14. How do you know you have leukemia?

Leukemia can become evident in many different ways. In fact, some patients have no symptoms at all, and the only reason the disease is diagnosed is because of routine blood testing. For example, at a routine physical, a blood test called a complete blood count (CBC) might be performed (see Question 16), and it might indicate that the white count is high or possibly even low. Alternatively, the platelet count might be depressed, as is common in acute leukemias. Finally, there may be signs of anemia in the CBC, which also could lead to a further examination of the bone marrow.

Many patients, however, *do* have symptoms that eventually bring them to a physician. Unfortunately, the symptoms are relatively vague and nonspecific. For example, generalized fatigue is very common because of the anemia that many patients experience with leukemia. Infection that is not very responsive to antibiotics or that simply persists for a longer than usual period of time is also a sign of leukemia. Abnormal bleeding may also be noticed. For instance, there may be bleeding in the gums from a low platelet count, or there may be diffuse swelling of the gums in addition to bleeding, which is common in acute myelomonocytic leukemia, one of the common types of AML. Small red dots may appear on the lower parts of the legs or in the oral cavity; these little dots are known as **petechiae** and are due to a very low platelet

Petechiae

Small red dots on the skin as a result of a very low platelet count.

count. Excessive bruising may be noticed, also due to a low platelet count. Some patients experience a feeling of fullness in their abdomen, especially after eating, due to an enlarged spleen. This is particularly common in CML. Children sometimes experience swollen lymph nodes and perhaps sore joints in association with ALL. The best general advice is to seek medical attention if you have severe fatigue, abnormal bleeding, or infections that persist. A full examination, including blood work, can usually disclose whether leukemia may be present. A final diagnosis is usually made after bone marrow biopsy and aspiration (see Question 17) are performed. *Remember that the overwhelming majority of people who have the symptoms of fatigue and a persistent infection **will not** turn out to have leukemia.* However, it is such a serious disease to go undiagnosed that it needs to be considered early in the differential diagnosis of these general complaints.

The best general advice is to seek medical attention if you have severe fatigue, abnormal bleeding, or infections that persist.

Pulling all of this information together, here is what happens when a patient is suspected of having leukemia. If the symptoms and some initial blood tests indicate that leukemia may be present, a careful physical examination and a more complete panel of blood tests will be performed, as will a bone marrow aspiration and biopsy. Samples of the marrow (and possibly the blood as well) will be studied by **flow cytometry** (a test done of cancerous tissues that shows the aggressiveness of a **tumor**, which is an abnormal tissue, swelling, or mass) and cytogenetic analysis (see Question 18), and the microscopic appearance of the leukemia cells will be examined. The results received from all of this testing can take days to weeks to accumulate. At this point, the precise diagnosis of the type and the subtype of leukemia can be made. This now

Flow cytometry

A test performed on cancerous tissues that shows the aggressiveness of the tumor.

Tumor

An abnormal tissue, swelling, or mass; may be either benign or malignant.

permits the next step, which is treatment. This will all be explained more fully below in subsequent questions.

15. What is neutropenia?

Neutropenia refers to a very low level of one of the important white blood cells, the neutrophil. The neutrophil, also known as the polymorphonuclear leukocyte, is a specialized type of white blood cell that protects us from bacterial and fungal pathogens (agents that cause infection). The neutrophil is able to engulf (phagocytose) bacteria that may or may not be coated with antibodies. This protective function is extremely effective at allowing a person to be free of infections caused by bacteria or fungi that are widespread in the environment. For example, bacteria, some of which could cause disease, heavily colonize the mouth and gastrointestinal tract. If defenses are down, they can enter into the bloodstream and cause serious, life-threatening infection. Normally, the neutrophil is situated in the tissues or in the bloodstream in a way that enables it to be the first line of defense against such invasion.

Severe neutropenia is a concentration of neutrophils in the blood of less than 500 cells per cubic millimeter (mm^3) of blood, which is about 20% of normal levels. Generally, there are approximately 2500 neutrophils per mm^3 of blood. When the neutrophil count is less than 500 per mm^3, the rate of bacterial and fungal infections is dramatically higher than when the count is above that number. Because the leukemia itself or the chemotherapy used to treat the leukemia is frequently associated with low neutrophil counts, neutropenia is common in patients with leukemia. Therefore, special

Neutropenia
A condition in which the body is depleted of important disease-fighting white blood cells.

Facts About Leukemia

consideration needs to be given for the patient's protection. A **neutropenic diet** (one that is low in microbes, meaning no fresh fruits and vegetables, or sushi and other raw meats, which might transmit infectious agents, such as bacteria, fungi, or parasites) is important because the ingestion of microscopic amounts of bacteria in salads and fresh fruits may lead to more virulent strains of bacteria. These bacteria ordinarily would be contained by the neutrophil, but when neutrophil levels are low, this function is lost, leading to potentially deadly infections. Secondly, in many situations, a patient is treated **prophylactically** with antibiotics to prevent disease or infection. The use of prophylactic antibiotics is not ideal, because this sometimes promotes the generation of resistant strains of bacteria or fungi. However, prophylactic antibiotics are generally useful in the neutropenic patient, who is particularly at risk for infection.

16. What is a CBC?

A test you will undergo frequently is a blood test called a **complete blood count** (**CBC**). This is the most important blood test for monitoring your leukemia and its response to treatment. A CBC provides the very useful and vital information concerning the levels of the three major blood cells, the red blood cells, the white blood cells, and the platelets (see Questions 1 and 9). You may see the results of your blood tests on a laboratory report, which can be confusing because a fairly large number of results are reported, giving one the impression that each is an individual test. In reality, the important numbers are the *WBC* (white blood count), the *hct* (the hematocrit, meaning the percentage of red blood cells in the blood), the *hgb* (the concentration of hemoglobin in the blood, which is very tightly correlated with the hct, so your doctor may just quote one of these numbers to you), and the *platelet* count. If you are puzzled by the numbers on your laboratory report, just ask your doctor or nurse to explain them to you.

When you are first diagnosed with leukemia, the doctor may obtain CBCs from you frequently, perhaps weekly or twice weekly, depending on the counts that are obtained. For example, if your platelet or red blood cell counts are low enough to raise the question of the need for blood or platelet transfusions (replacement of blood cells or platelets in the bloodstream when a person's own bone marrow is unable to do so), the frequency of blood draws will be higher. If your veins are in good condition, this should not be difficult. However, some patients have more problems, and their blood draws will require an experienced lab technician. Usually, before starting intense chemotherapy for acute leukemia or before a bone marrow transplantation, the patient will have a semi-permanent venous **catheter** surgically placed into one of the large veins under the collarbone. Blood can be removed from this catheter for tests. In addition, medications and transfusions can be delivered through this intravenous catheter. This eliminates the need for repeated needle sticks in your veins, making the treatment process virtually painless for you, and far easier for the nurses to complete. The actual catheter can sometimes be easily infected, so daily inspection and dressing changes are essential. Once the treatments are over, the frequency of CBCs and other blood tests will become less frequent. The catheter can be removed in a same-day procedure

Catheter

Device placed surgically beneath the skin to facilitate the frequent infusion of medications and/or other treatments.

Port-a-cath

A device surgically implanted under the skin, usually on the chest, that enters a large blood vessel and is used to deliver medication, chemotherapy, and blood products and also is used to obtain blood samples.

Bone marrow biopsy and aspiration

A procedure in which a needle is inserted into the center of a bone, usually the hip, to remove a small amount of bone marrow for microscopic examination.

Hematologist

A specialist who treats patients with malignancies (and other diseases) of the blood.

Oncologist

A physician who specializes in cancer treatment.

when it no longer is needed as part of ongoing therapy. In some settings, the device is called a **Port-a-cath**.

17. What is a bone marrow biopsy/aspiration? Is it painful?

A **bone marrow biopsy/aspiration**, usually performed by a **hematologist** (specialist in treating diseases, including malignancies, of the blood) or an **oncologist** (specialist in oncology, the science dealing with the physical, chemical, and biologic properties and features of cancer, including causes, the disease process, and treatment), involves inserting a needle into the cavity of the pelvis bone to withdraw samples of bone marrow and the surrounding bone. It is performed under local anesthesia similar to what a dentist would use to work on a tooth. First, a needle is inserted into the bone marrow cavity to allow a small amount of liquid marrow (which looks like blood) to be withdrawn. After this needle is removed, a second needle is used to remove a small (about half an inch long) cylinder of bone, which then undergoes pathology testing (biopsy). The procedure takes 30–45 minutes and is often considered uncomfortable. Of course, some patients may experience more pain than others from this procedure, depending on their own sensitivity to pain, the skill of the person doing the procedure, and any technical difficulties encountered during the test. The purpose of the test is to examine cells in the bone marrow carefully under the microscope in order to determine whether any abnormalities exist. When leukemia is suspected, for example, based on an abnormality in the blood cells, it is necessary to do a bone marrow aspiration. This procedure may be repeated during leukemia treatment to monitor the progress of therapy. For example, after induction (initial) chemotherapy for leukemia, the bone marrow aspiration may be repeated to demonstrate that normal cells have repopulated the bone marrow and that the leukemia cells have been eliminated.

18. What are chromosomes/cytogenetics?

Every cell in the human body, with the exception of the red blood cells, contains a nucleus, which in turn contains chromosomes. The **chromosomes** are large, complex structures that contain DNA and proteins. The **DNA** (one of two nucleic acids found in the nucleus of all cells) is organized into genes, which code for proteins that are necessary for all functionality of the cell and, ultimately, the individual. The anatomy of the chromosome can be studied by performing a clinical test called "karyotyping" or **cytogenetic analysis**. This analysis refers to a procedure whereby cells, taken from either the blood or the bone marrow, are cultured in a specialized laboratory in such a way that the dividing cells are arrested in the middle of their division. At this time, the chromosomes have organized themselves into structures that can be seen under the microscope with appropriate staining. In this manner, the number and the exact characteristics of the chromosomes can be seen. Normally, there are 46 chromosomes in each cell. A female has two "X" chromosomes and a male has an "X" and a "Y" chromosome. The remaining pairs of chromosomes do not differ according to gender. That is, chromosomes 1 through 22 are the same in a male or a female. In malignant cells, such as leukemia cells and lymphoma cells, unique alterations are observed on a regular basis in the chromosomes. Thus, cytogenetic analysis yields important information regarding the exact nature of the genetic defect

Facts About Leukemia

Chromosomes

Large complex structures that contain DNA and proteins.

DNA

One of two nucleic acids (the other is RNA) found in the nucleus of all cells. DNA contains genetic information on cell growth, division and cell function.

Cytogenetic analysis

A procedure whereby cells, taken from either the blood or the bone marrow, are cultured in a specialized laboratory in such a way that the dividing cells are arrested in the middle of their division. The structure of the chromosomes can then be stained and visualized by a microscope.

31

that is associated with a given patient's leukemia. This, in turn, leads to important information regarding the patient's prognosis. For example, certain cytogenetic abnormalities, such as **translocations**, which means that one piece of a chromosome moves to another chromosome, are associated with different prognoses after chemotherapy. Some abnormalities favor a good outcome—that is, chances are good that the patient will survive. Thus, the identification of one of these favorable cytogenetic abnormalities can lead to the application of the treatment that offers the best chance of survival without the excess risk posed by perhaps a more aggressive treatment. Conversely, certain cytogenetic abnormalities have been associated with a very poor outcome. In such an event, a physician may use such information to consider not treating a patient aggressively, if the situation warrants this decision. For example, an elderly or infirm patient may be counseled to have supportive care or only "mild" chemotherapy if the prognosis is considered extremely poor, because chances are good that the treatment would not work, and the patient would suffer a lower quality of life for no reason. The identification of these chromosomal changes has also been useful in leading to advances in the treatment of leukemia and in understanding more fundamental aspects of the biology of leukemia. It is considered routine to perform cytogenetic analysis on a newly diagnosed leukemia so that the prognosis can be determined.

In CML, a very characteristic and universal cytogenetic abnormality is observed. Under the microscope, one can see a very small piece of chromosomal material, originally called the **Philadelphia chromosome**, which is a translocation of part of chromosome 9 to chromosome 22 and vice versa. This 9:22 translocation

Translocation

The movement of one piece of chromosome to another chromosome.

Philadelphia-chromosome

The abnormal chromosome found in patients with CML.

is diagnostic of CML; in other words, if the translocation is present, the doctor can be absolutely certain that the patient has CML.

The identification of the genes involved has also allowed the discovery of the **pathogenesis** (the origin and development) of this disease. The genes code for a recently identified protein referred to as "bcr/abl," which is responsible for the excess cellular division observed in CML. The "abl" portion of the molecule is an enzyme that acts to drive cellular proliferation. Recently, a designer drug was created to block the activity of this enzyme. This drug, recently approved as Gleevec (see Question 22), inhibits this enzyme, which is unique to CML.

Pathogenesis
The origin and development of a disease.

Cytogenetic analysis in ALL is useful in demonstrating that a large proportion (33%) of adult patients with ALL have the Philadelphia chromosome in their cells. This is an important observation because the prognosis of patients with this type of ALL is quite poor compared with those without the translocation. This information thus has led to the use of bone marrow transplantation to patients with ALL who have the Philadelphia chromosome; this treatment has been found to cure a substantial portion of people.

Patients with CLL frequently have an extra chromosome 12, referred to as "trisomy 12." This has been associated with a worse prognosis.

Cytogenetics are routinely performed at diagnosis in the acute leukemias and in suspected cases of CML. Cytogenetics may then be performed at different phases of treatment to document the elimination of these abnormal cells.

Facts About Leukemia

19. What is immunophenotyping?

Leukemia cells, like all blood cells, display numerous protein, carbohydrate, and lipid molecules on the outer surface of the cell. These various molecules, sometimes referred to as **antigens**, are often important components of the cell for signaling, attaching to surfaces, and as docking sites for **growth factors** for the leukemia or normal cells. **Immunophenotyping** refers to a laboratory test whereby these antigens can be measured on the surface of the leukemia cell. The purpose of this test is to determine the type of leukemia that exists in a given patient. For example, AML expresses antigens that are characteristic of normal granulocytes and monocytes, whereas ALL has the same antigens expressed by normal lymphocytes. A more refined application of this technique also involves identifying an abnormal immunophenotype, which can be used to monitor the progress of treatment. For example, a leukemia cell may express myeloid antigens predominantly but may also express a lymphoid antigen; however, this is not a normal situation. This mixed phenotype may then be monitored during treatment by repeating the immunophenotyping. The testing can be performed on blood cells as well as on bone marrow cells.

Immunopheno-typing

A laboratory test whereby antigens can be measured on the surface of the leukemia cell.

PART THREE

Treatment

How is leukemia treated?

What is chemotherapy?

How does my doctor decide
which chemotherapy to give?

More ...

20. How is leukemia treated?

Leukemia is a systemic disease, which means that any treatment administered must be able to reach all parts of the body. There is no role for surgery and a very, very limited role for **radiation therapy** (treatment with high-energy x-rays to destroy cancer cells). Thus, therapy for leukemia consists of the administration of chemotherapy. Chemotherapy is more or less defined as therapy with **cytotoxic drugs**, that is, drugs that are able to kill leukemia cells. A large number of drugs that are specific for the different forms of leukemia are used to treat it. Other approaches to the treatment of leukemia include immunotherapy, which involves using monoclonal antibodies, certain types of cells, or certain biologic molecules referred to as cytokines, such as interleukin-2 (see Question 28). Many of these therapies are investigational at this time.

A patient with acute leukemia who has achieved a complete remission but has a high probability of relapse, may undergo a **hematopoietic stem cell transplantation** (provision of new stem cells to the patient) to improve the odds of staying in complete remission (see Question 33).

21. What is chemotherapy?

Chemotherapy refers to the administration of drugs that are capable of killing cancer cells, or at least retarding their growth. These drugs are manufactured by the pharmaceutical industry and are regulated by the FDA, whose approval is required for their commercial use. Chemotherapy drugs may be given **orally** (by mouth, e.g., Gleevec, hydroxyurea), **intravenously** (injected into a vein, e.g., cytosine arabinoside, flu-

Radiation therapy

Treatment with high-energy x-rays to destroy cancer cells.

Cytotoxic

Drugs that can kill cancer cells. Usually refers to drugs used in chemotherapy treatments.

Hematopoietic stem cell transplantation

The process by which new stem cells are introduced into a patient.

Chemotherapy

Treatment of cancer by use of chemicals; often uses two or more chemicals to achieve maximum kill of tumor cells. Usually refers to drugs used to treat cancer.

Orally

Taken by mouth.

Intravenously

Entering the body through a vein.

darabine), or even **subcutaneously** (injected under the skin, e.g., L-asparaginase). Chemotherapy has been the mainstay of leukemia treatment for decades. Recently, biologic agents, such as monoclonal antibodies (see Question 27), are increasingly used either alone or in conjunction with conventional chemotherapy.

Table 2 lists some of the medications used to treat leukemia. The exact treatment of an individual takes into consideration many factors. There is no single drug or combination that is considered so "standard" that every doctor uses it. The names of medications may be confusing—drugs can be referred to by their trade (brand) name or by their "generic" name. Furthermore, sometimes an abbreviated slang-like use will be employed. For example, the drug cytosine arabinoside (generic) may be called cytarabine (another generic), Cytosar (trade), or ara-c (slang). Obviously, this can be confusing to the patient. When in doubt about what you are hearing, please ask your doctor to clarify!

22. What is Gleevec?

Gleevec is the trade name for a chemical called imatinib mesylate. In the clinical trial phase of its development, this drug was also called STI–571. Gleevec is a small chemical molecule that was developed to specifically inhibit the enzyme that is overactive in patients with CML. The malignant cells in CML have an abnormal protein that has heightened activity of an enzyme known as tyrosine kinase. Gleevec inhibits the enzyme so that its activity is suppressed in the CML cells. Doctors and patients alike were pleasantly surprised by the findings that this oral drug could give rise to remissions in CML. At one level, the remission

Subcutaneously
Injected under the skin.

Treatment

Gleevec
Oral chemotherapy agent approved for use in patients with CML.

Table 2   Medications Commonly Used for Treating Different Leukemias

Leukemia	Commonly Used Drugs	Also known as:
AML	Cytarabine	Ara-C, Cytosar-U
	Idarubicin	Idamycin
	Daunorubicin	Cerubidine
	Mitoxantrone	Novantrone
	VP–16	Etoposide
	Gemtuzumab ozogamicin	Mylotarg
ALL	Cyclophosphamide	Cytoxan
	Vincristine	Oncovin
	Prednisone	Deltasone
	Daunorubicin	Cerubidine
	L–Asparaginase	Oncaspar
	Cytarabine	Ara-C, Cytosar-U
	Methotrexate	Amethopeterin, Folex
	6-Mercaptopurine	Purinethol
	6-Thioguanine	Tabloid
CML	STI–571, Imatinib mesylate	Gleevec, Glivec
	Hydroxyurea	Hydrea
	Interferon alpha	Intron A
CLL	Fludarabine	Fludara
	Cyclophosphamide	Cytoxan
	Prednisone	Deltasone
	Chlorambucil	Leukeran
	Alemtuzumab	Campath

is called **hematologic**, meaning that the blood counts return to normal. More importantly, some patients experience a disappearance of the Philadelphia chromosome, which means that there is even less likelihood of the disease coming right back.

Finally, some patients even achieve **molecular remissions**, in which special tests that can amplify very small numbers of cells can be used to see whether the disease has been totally eradicated. The FDA approved Gleevec in 2001 for CML patients. It has been quite safe, with the only serious side effects being fluid retention, rash, hemorrhage, bleeding, and kidney and liver toxicity, and those in only a small number of patients. Most patients tolerate Gleevec very well without any side effects. Because the drug has been in use for only the past couple of years, it is impossible to predict its long-term effectiveness. Some believe that patients with the most profound decrease in their malignant cells (whose disease cannot be detected even with molecular techniques) may experience long-term survival without recurrence of the disease. Patients who have more accelerated or blastic forms of CML also respond, but their responses are temporary. Thus, this drug is increasingly used to treat the more aggressive forms of CML temporarily while arrangements are attempted for a bone marrow transplantation.

The role of bone marrow transplantation for patients in the first chronic phase of CML is controversial. Most physicians would still say that if an HLA-matched sibling donor is available for a patient under the age of 50, allogeneic transplantation should be strongly considered because it is the only known curative therapy for this disease. For patients over 50 years of age, a trial of

Hematologic remission

Remission defined by the blood counts' return to normal.

Molecular remission

Remission defined by analysis of small numbers of cells that indicate that a disease is totally eradicated.

Treatment

39

Gleevec may be indicated first to demonstrate whether the patient responds to this drug. If the patient does respond, long-term maintenance with Gleevec would be the best choice. It is too soon to say how long a patient needs to continue receiving Gleevec therapy—it may or may not be a life-long therapy.

23. What is ATRA? How would arsenic be used?

ATRA stands for all-*trans*-retinoic acid, a drug whose structure is related to that of vitamin A. Amazingly, this drug, which was first studied by Chinese doctors, induces the relatively uncommon form of AML known as promyelocytic leukemia (10% of AML) to differentiate into normal end-stage white blood cells. This means that the leukemic cells become like normal white blood cells, so the effects of leukemia disappear. Another bonus is that this drug is given orally. However, because ATRA alone does not produce long-lasting remissions, current treatment protocols combine ATRA with conventional anti-AML drugs, such as cytosine arabinoside.

Arsenic trioxide, also discovered by Chinese scientists, is able to induce differentiation in promyelocytic leukemia cells as well. It is now approved by the FDA for use in patients with relapsed promyelocytic leukemia, and it is also being tested in clinical trials against other types of cancer.

24. How does my doctor decide which chemotherapy to give?

This is a very complicated question, and standards of care for leukemia are evolving continually. A large amount of clinical research has gone into the creation of the current treatment protocols. However, because none of the current treatments are perfect, clinical research and clinical trials continue to seek better treatments. In addition, new **pharmaceuticals** (medications) are always being developed, which allows the introduction of these new agents into treatment protocols. So how your doctor decides to treat your leukemia has a lot to do with who your doctor is, the type of medical center in which you are being treated, the specifics of your illness, your age, and other potential health problems. Relatively standard treatments for each of the major leukemias do exist, but there is constant evolution in the treatments because the "perfect" treatment that can cure everyone has not yet been discovered.

You might be offered entry into a clinical trial at a major medical center (see Question 29). The clinical trial has been carefully considered and reviewed by multiple levels of scrutiny and is believed to offer the best chance of remission and long-term survival. However, the requirements for entry on a clinical trial are fairly rigid. Therefore, it is not uncommon for a patient to be treated with a standard regimen instead of being entered into a clinical trial. This is where the experience of your physician and his or her institution are relevant. For example, an institution may be very comfortable giving one form of therapy, while another institution may be comfortable with a different form of therapy, which they believe is equally effective. This can be difficult for the patient to sort out and understand. Further decision making hinges on your physician's assessment of your disease and your overall condition. For instance, an older patient with other problems, such as heart failure or coronary artery disease, may be treated less aggressively than a young

Pharmaceuticals
Medications that are continuously being developed for future patient care.

Treatment

41

Prognostic factors

Factors that help to determine the severity of a disease.

It is not unreasonable to ask your physician to explain his or her thinking regarding the choice of treatment.

Protocol

A schedule of selected drugs and treatment time intervals known to be effective against a certain cancer.

Gene therapy

Investigational treatment of disease by the introduction of new genetic material into cells in order to modify their DNA.

patient with no pre-existing illness. Finally, the use of **prognostic factors,** such as cytogenetics, may direct treatment to be more or less aggressive. It is not unreasonable to ask your physician to explain to you his or her thinking regarding the choice of treatments offered to you for any form of leukemia.

The **protocols** (schedules of drugs and treatment) for treating the different types of leukemia vary. Protocols are constantly changing, and new drugs are becoming available constantly. However, with new medications can come undiscovered challenges. Each person has different reactions, because each of our chemistries is unique. Even though the chemotherapy drugs are generally safe, there is an unavoidable risk of side effects, and you should be made aware of potential side effects that may occur either immediately or later. You should also inquire whether there are any interactions between your chemotherapy drugs and any other medications you may be taking.

25. What is gene therapy?

Gene therapy is a term applied to a wide range of research efforts to introduce new genetic material into cells in order to modify their DNA. There have been some intriguing early successes in the use of this therapeutic approach for patients with immune deficiency states and hemophilia. However, in general, this is still a very investigational form of therapy. Applications in leukemia would include efforts to render leukemia cells more antigenic (meaning foreign) to the immune system of the patient. Other efforts might be to introduce genes into the chromosomes that decrease the proliferative rate of leukemia cells. Currently, there are no clinically applicable gene therapy approaches for most patients with leukemia, and this remains an experimental approach.

26. What is anti-sense therapy?

This is another emerging but investigational therapy for a variety of diseases, including leukemia and other forms of cancer. The basic idea of **anti-sense therapy** is to block the production of a key protein involved in the progression of a cancer using specially crafted strings of DNA that can get into cells and block the corresponding RNA that makes the protein of interest. The protein that the cancer cell makes is made by the "sense" strand of RNA. The "anti-sense" is the mirror image of the "sense" strand, and is able to neutralize it. For example, leukemia cells have an excess of a protein called bcl-2 that blocks the normal death of a cell. Blocking bcl-2 production leads to death of leukemia cells in the laboratory. Clinical trials of bcl-2 anti-sense are being conducted to determine whether a therapeutic benefit can be achieved in patients with AML and other cancers.

Anti-sense therapy

Emerging investigational therapy for various diseases that blocks protein production.

27. What is a monoclonal antibody?

A **monoclonal antibody** is a highly specialized antibody that is usually produced initially by immunizing a mouse with an antigen of interest. The spleen from the mouse is then fused with a cell type that lends the property of immortality to the lymphocytes in the spleen. This cell, known as a hybridoma, produces an unlimited quantity of a single antibody molecule from the lymphocyte. This antibody is known as a monoclonal antibody (which is an antibody with only one specificity or

Monoclonal antibody

Antibody that specifically binds to a particular molecule on the surface of a certain type of leukemia or other cancer.

Treatment

antigen). Research scientists have employed this process for over 20 years since its discovery by the Nobel prize winners Koehler and Milstein. Recently, because of the ability to produce human monoclonal antibodies, the human forms have replaced the mouse antibodies in clinical trials. These human monoclonal antibodies can be produced such that they specifically bind to a particular molecule on the surface of a certain type of leukemia or other cancer. Thus, monoclonal antibodies are available to antigens expressed on leukemia cells that either are now approved for clinical use or are under active study in clinical trials. For example, Mylotarg, a monoclonal antibody with a chemotherapy drug attached to it, was recently approved for the treatment of AML. Another monoclonal antibody, Campath, was also recently approved for the treatment of CLL. Many more monoclonal antibodies are under active study that hopefully will be available for wide use in the future. It is expected that the optimal use of monoclonal antibodies will be in combination with standard chemotherapy agents, providing therapies that are more potent without being more toxic.

28. What is immunotherapy?

Immunotherapy

Treatment that stimulates the body's own defense mechanisms to combat diseases such as cancer.

Immunotherapy is a general term referring to the use of the immune system to treat disease. There has been an interest in immunotherapy for a long time, based on theory and animal studies that the immune system itself can control tumor growth. However, most immunotherapeutic approaches to the treatment of leukemia remain investigational. That said, there are now a number of emerging immunotherapies that seem to be effective. In the treatment of leukemia, immunotherapy may mean the use of monoclonal antibodies, cytokines such as interleukin-2, or cells such as T lymphocytes and natural killer cells. Immunotherapy is considered a biologic therapy because it harnesses normal components of our bodies in an effort to direct these elements to help eliminate the leukemia.

29. What is a clinical trial?

A **clinical trial** is a study examining the safety and effectiveness of a treatment of an illness. There are many kinds of clinical trials, and therefore it is important to understand the distinction between them.

A *phase I* clinical trial is the earliest testing of either a new drug or possibly the use of an established drug, but for a new disease. For example, a drug may already be approved for treating a certain form of leukemia, but it may be tested for the treatment of a different form of leukemia in a phase I study that is trying to determine the safety and the best dose of the drug for that particular leukemia.

A *phase II* study typically involves the use of a particular drug at a fixed dose, which has been already established in a phase I study to be safe and possibly effective. The phase II study attempts to determine the effectiveness of the drug used in a standard manner in a larger number of patients.

A *phase III* study typically compares the activity of one drug or combination of drugs with the activity of another drug or combination of drugs, both of which are already established as having activity in a particular disease. The phase III study may determine

Treatment

Clinical trial

A specific treatment protocol that is designed to test the effectiveness and safety of a drug or combination of drugs, or other therapies, in the treatment of a disease.

45

whether a new drug or combination of drugs that has recently been developed can be more effective than the established treatment for that particular leukemia. Clinical trials are sometimes referred to as *investigational* or *experimental*. These terms sometimes cause confusion, especially when it comes to payment for treatment by insurance companies; many insurance companies have clauses that disallow the use of experimental treatments for their members. However, in the treatment of leukemia, a drug may be used that has shown promise but has not yet received FDA approval. Thus, an insurance company may state that the treatment is experimental and may therefore disallow it, even when the community of physicians has determined that this may be the best new drug for leukemia in some time. An insurance company may even deem it experimental when an FDA-approved drug is included in a clinical trial if it is used in a slightly different dose or schedule, again with the goal of improving outcomes.

Experts in leukemia treatment are always trying to improve the outcomes of treatment, but they sometimes get caught in a bind with the third-party payers of the treatment. Frequently, when truly experimental agents, such as new drugs, are being used, the sponsoring pharmaceutical company pays for all elements of the treatment that are considered investigational. This would include the drug itself and any additional testing that would be performed specifically because the patient was in a clinical trial. Certain legislation has been enacted to mandate that insurance companies pay for treatment that occurs in clinical trials, recognizing that advances in treatment can come only from widespread participation in clinical trials. It is notable that in pediatric populations, approximately 95% of patients in the United States are treated in national-level clinical trials. In contrast, only 5% of adult patients are enrolled in clinical trials in the United States. Studies have shown that outcomes in patient care are improved when patients are treated in clinical trials, presumably because of the intense scrutiny involved when the patient is treated in a clinical trial. Clinical trial monitoring is very intense and rigorous, and this increased attention to the details of management, quality of life, follow-up, and compliance with treatment are probable reasons for improved outcomes in clinical trials.

30. What are study drugs? Are there any promising new drugs in development?

Clinical trials may consist of studies of new agents. Therefore, a study drug is a new pharmacologic agent that is being tested for a new therapeutic activity. The usual course of events is that new agents are discovered in academic or pharmaceutical laboratories that have activity on leukemia cells in the laboratory. For example, a drug may be identified that kills leukemia cells in the test tube. After appropriate safety testing in small animal strains and possibly even in primates (that is, monkeys and apes, which are the animals most closely related to humans), the drug is then introduced to patients who have advanced disease. After efficacy and safety are shown, the drug is then pursued in more widespread clinical trials.

As of the publication of this book, several new drugs are in development for the treatment of leukemia. Current thinking is that successful drugs need to target the abnormal proteins in leukemia cells that are responsible for making the cells grow in such an uncontrolled manner. Two of these are investigational drugs that target selected biochemical pathways in leukemia cells that are abnormally activated to promote leukemia cell growth. These drugs target the enzyme farnesyl transferase and the cell surface protein FLT–3, two proteins involved in the control of cell division. In addition, a class of drugs is under study that can inhibit the enzyme histone deacetylase, resulting in the removal of gene-silencing molecules that somehow contribute to leukemia cell growth. Other targets for anti-leukemia therapy include angiogenesis inhibitors, including thalidomide, SU5416, and monoclonal antibodies to vascular endothelial growth factor, with the hope that attacking the blood supply to leukemia cells will starve them to death.

Ask your doctor about what clinical trials are available.

These approaches are all investigational. Some of the drugs may work, others won't. In addition, certain drugs may work on certain leukemias and not others. You should ask your doctor about what clinical trials are available at his or her institution or practice, as well as where trials of new agents are being conducted if not at his or her institution or practice.

31. What determines who is eligible for a study?

A clinical trial has strict eligibility and exclusion criteria for entry into the study; the exact diagnosis, subtypes of leukemia, age of the patient, history of previous treatment, history of other illnesses, and a myriad of other issues are addressed in these criteria. However, the physician treating the patient or the patient must first be aware of the clinical trials. This crucial step is often lacking and is the reason why many patients are not enrolled in clinical trials. Once it is recognized that a patient may be eligible for a particular clinical trial, there are numerous support staff at large institutions or at clinical trial-oriented private practices that are available for screening patients for eligibility. In addition to obvious factors, such as diagnosis, age, and type of leukemia, a number of laboratory tests may be performed to determine that the overall health of the patient is suited for the study. The process of **informed consent** is always utilized. This means that the patient is told explicitly what the elements of the clinical trial are and what the risks and benefits to the patient may be. The patient may withdraw from treatment at any time, because participation in the study is completely voluntary. The patient signs an agreement to the terms of the study. This so-called consent form is then part of the patient's medical record.

Informed Consent

Process of explaining to the patient of all risks and complications of a procedure or treatment before it is done. Most informed consents are written and signed by the patient or a legal representative.

Treatment

PART FOUR

Blood and Marrow Stem Cell Transplantation

What is a stem cell?

What is stem cell transplantation?

More . . .

32. What is a stem cell?

Stem cell

A primitive type of cell from which all cells of a given organ or tissue arise.

Tissue

A collection of similar cells. There are four basic types of tissues in the body epithelial, connective, muscle, and nerve.

Hematopoietic stem cell

Referring to its ability to make all the cellular elements of the blood.

Broadly defined, a **stem cell** is a type of cell in the body that can continuously replenish the cells of that particular **tissue** (a tissue is a collection of similar cells). One can think of it as a seed that gives rise to the remainder of cells in that particular tissue. This implies that there are organ-specific stem cells. For example, there is a type of stem cell that resides in the bone marrow that is capable of giving rise to all of the blood cells that are first formed in the bone marrow and then travel to the blood. This cell is referred to as a **hematopoietic stem cell**. There appear to be stem cells in other organs as well, that are specific for these organs. For instance, there may be a liver (hepatic) stem cell, a muscle stem cell, and a neural stem cell. There are also intriguing observations suggesting that stem cells from one tissue may actually still retain some properties of giving rise to cells of another tissue under certain conditions. This is referred to as "stem cell plasticity." A general property of stem cells is that they can renew themselves. Thus, when a stem cell divides, it replenishes itself, but it also gives rise to a daughter cell that begins the process of differentiation into the tissues in which it resides. Stem cells are rare in any tissue. They make up no more than .01% of the total cells in the bone marrow, for example. They can be defined with certain cell-surface markers and by their abilities to make colonies of blood cells in the laboratory. The bone marrow stem cell can migrate into the blood. These are the cells that are transplanted in a bone marrow transplant.

33. What is stem cell transplantation?

The term *stem cell transplantation* has crept into the jargon of medicine. Previously, these treatments were referred to as "bone marrow transplants" or BMTs. In a BMT, the goal is to transplant the hematopoietic stem cell. In general, **stem cell transplantation** is the process by which stem cells are infused into a patient. The patient is generally prepared for the procedure by administration of very high doses of chemotherapy in a hospital setting over a period of several days, with careful monitoring and adjustment of the chemotherapy. Before receiving chemotherapy, the patient usually has an indwelling catheter placed (see Question 16), allowing for easier administration of chemotherapy, blood drawing, blood transfusions, and antibiotic therapy.

Stem cell transplantation

The process by which new stem cells are infused into a patient.

Recovery can be slow because the stem cells have to begin producing blood cells again. At this time (a period of weeks), the patient is most fragile and is at high risk for infection. Extreme caution and careful management of food, diet, dust, and exposure to elements, as well as limiting of visitors, will enhance the patient's ability to successfully navigate this difficult period until the blood counts recover.

34. Who should have a stem cell transplant?

This is a complicated question that requires considerable deliberation and judgment by the patient and the doctor alike. Stem cell transplants have been commonly used in the management of the acute leukemias and CML. That said, only a small fraction of patients with these forms of leukemia end up getting a stem cell transplant. The goal of transplantation is usually cure. Those making the decision must consider the odds that a cure could be achieved by conventional chemotherapy, compared with the odds that a transplant will achieve that goal. Several factors are considered, including the age of the patient, the molecular characteristics of the disease, and the availability of a suitable stem cell donor. To some extent, the decision to undergo transplantation can be subjected to objective criteria that can even be reduced to an algorithm. For example, a patient with AML under the age of 60 who has an HLA-matched sibling donor (see Question 46) and whose disease has features that predict a poor prognosis with standard therapy would most likely be offered allogeneic stem cell transplantation. On the other hand, if the patient's leukemia has "good risk features," meaning that his or her prognosis looks favorable, allogeneic stem cell transplantation might not offer an increased chance of cure, and therefore, the increased risk of transplantation is not warranted. As new information is generated from clinical research studies, the decision of who should undergo transplantation requires careful and considered judgment. Ask your doctor to explain why you should or shouldn't be referred for a blood or bone marrow stem cell transplant.

35. What is the difference between autologous and allogeneic transplantation?

Autologous stem cell transplantation involves the use of cells from the patient's own body. Blood stem cells are generally collected by use of a special intravenous catheter placed directly either into a vein in the arm or under the collarbone. Autologous stem cell transplantations are commonly used in leukemia, lymphoma, and myeloma. The patient must be in remission so that stem cells that are not contaminated with cancer cells can be collected. Allogeneic stem cell transplantation involves the use of cells from someone other than the patient. Typically, a sibling donor who is matched at histocompatibility antigens (see Question 46) is called on to donate either bone marrow or blood stem cells to be used to infuse into the patient, who has received chemotherapy or radiotherapy to prepare them for the stem cell transplant. Recently, doctors are trying less "intense" chemotherapy or radiation doses in an effort to reduce the toxicity of allogeneic stem cell transplantation. You may hear these infusions referred to as "mini" transplants, reduced intensity transplants, or non-myeloablative transplants—all terms referring to the same concept. Occasionally, a patient has an identical twin who could act as a donor. The advantage of this situation is that the donor and the patient are fully matched for all important tissue antigens. Thus, there is no graft-versus-host reaction (see Questions 63–65) or rejection. The only disadvantage is that there is also less of a graft-versus-leukemia effect (see Question 63), because the donor lymphocytes do not recognize any of the patient's leukemia cell antigens as foreign. This is most relevant for transplantations for CML. Unrelated donors that are well-matched with the patient are also used for allogeneic transplants.

Another form of unrelated donor cells is from umbilical cord blood, and there are numerous cord blood registries now that might have a suitably matched unit, stored frozen, already in the bank. There is much less experience with this form of transplant for adults, but the number of transplantations performed with umbilical cord blood is increasing. Allogeneic transplants are used in both acute and chronic leukemias.

36. How is it determined which one is appropriate for my care?

The decision on whether to perform autologous versus allogeneic transplantation is complicated. The first issue is whether there is a suitable **donor** (one who donates cells or marrow) for a particular patient. If there is not a sibling or closely related family member who is matched at the histocompatibility antigens (see Question 46), allogeneic stem cell transplantation is ruled out. An unrelated donor transplantation may be pursued, but given the higher rates of graft-versus-host disease (Questions 63–65) with this type of transplantation, it is limited to a younger population of patients—generally under 50, perhaps up to 60 years of age—with recently introduced reduced intensity preparative regimens for allogeneic transplants. Autologous transplantation may be used in some cases of acute leukemia, based on clinical trials that have shown the relative value of these transplants. The age of the patient is a factor in the decision of which type of transplantation to pursue, as are some of the characteristics of the disease. Of course, if there is not a suitable HLA-matched donor, then an autologous transplantation may be the only option for many patients.

Donor

One who donates blood stem cells or bone marrow for infusion into a patient.

37. How long after diagnosis should the transplant take place?

This, again, is a complex clinical decision. If an HLA-matched sibling is available for a patient with acute leukemia in first complete remission, there is evidence that proceeding to transplantation after achieving complete remission is often the best course of action. Ideally, the patient should have recovered fully from the effects of chemotherapy and not have any lingering side effects or infections before undergoing the bone marrow transplantation. If a decision had already been made not to do the transplantation in first remission and the patient eventually has a relapse, then transplantation should be strongly considered after a second remission is induced.

Transplants were formerly the treatment of choice in CML in the first year after diagnosis. The discovery of the new drug Gleevec has led many patients to try this drug first and forego transplantation unless a remission isn't achieved or they have a relapse.

38. What is total body irradiation (TBI)? Will I need to have it?

Allogeneic transplantation for AML, ALL, and CML often includes total body irradiation (TBI). There is an alternative regimen that involves drugs only. TBI means that the entire body is exposed to the same intensity of radiation. Radiation physicians and physicists carefully calculate the dose, so that the amount of radiation getting into every part of the body is approximately the same. This is important because leukemia cells can be dispersed throughout every capillary or blood vessel in the body, so it is necessary to irradiate the entire body to ensure that every leukemia cell has been irradiated.

39. What are immunosuppressive drugs and who is likely to need them?

Patients undergoing stem cell transplantation from a donor (allogeneic transplantation) require treatment with immunosuppressive drugs. This is because if the function of the patient's immune system is not suppressed, the transplanted donor cells would be immediately rejected. Immunosuppression allows the transplanted donor cells to survive and eventually develop the new bone marrow and immune system. Another reason that immunosuppressive drugs are used in this type of transplantation is that they decrease the possibility of graft versus host disease (see Questions 63–65). The immunosuppressive drugs decrease the aggressiveness of the newly developing immune system, which might react against the patient's tissues if the immunosuppressive drugs were not being given.

Many drugs are immunosuppressive; the most familiar immunosuppressive drug to many patients is prednisone, or its intravenous form, solumedrol. Dexamethasone is another variation of prednisone that is commonly used as immunosuppression. Other drugs often used, including cyclosporine (Neoral) and tacrolimus (FK–506, Prograf), are very selective inhibitors of T-lymphocyte (lymphocytes that directly attach themselves to virally infected or transformed cells to mediate their destruction) function, whereas prednisone has broader actions on a variety of cells and tissues in the body. The side effects of prednisone and its relatives are numerous and include high blood sugar, thinning of the bones, mood changes, and deterioration of muscle tissue. All of these side effects are dose and time dependent, meaning that if a patient has to receive high doses of the drug for a longer period of time, the side effects are much more likely to occur. On the other hand, if the drugs are used for a brief period of time, the side effects may be minimal. Side effects of cyclosporine and tacrolimus are somewhat different. These agents sometimes cause mild kidney failure, high blood pressure, and neurologic side effects, like visual changes and seizures. Again, these side effects, although serious, are uncommon, and they are dose and time dependent.

Another important side effect of immunosuppressive drugs is an increased incidence of infection. Because the immune system is depressed, patients are likely to develop any of the infections discussed earlier (see Question 56). Your doctors take this into consideration when using immunosuppressive drugs. They may place you on prophylactic antibiotics (therapy geared to *prevent* infection) to decrease the chance that an infection will develop. On balance, the benefits from these drugs far exceed the side effects.

40. Do I need to stay on immunosuppressive drugs for life?

The answer is generally "no." Usually, the patient's tolerance of the graft can develop in the first 6 to 12 months after transplant, leading to the opportunity to withdraw immune suppression. Occasionally, chronic graft-versus-host disease (see Question 62) may require prolonged immunosuppression, sometimes for life. The degree of immunosuppression can be quite variable between patients, ranging from very mild such as a small dose of prednisone, to more intense multidrug regimens.

41. When will I regain my new immune system after transplantation?

Immunodeficiency after stem cell transplantation is common and prolonged. In an HLA-matched sibling transplantation (see Question 46), the immune system generally returns to normal after approximately one year. In patients undergoing unrelated donor stem cell transplantation, the immunodeficiency may last for a longer period of time because the new T cells are not able to react to antigens as well in this situation.

42. What is the success rate of bone marrow transplantation?

People often want to know the answer to this general question, but it is difficult to give simple answers to this question. The main reason for this is that the answer differs for each type of leukemia, and it is also dependent on the age of the patient, the time in the history of the disease at which the transplantation is performed, and the type of transplantation performed. A very general answer is that approximately 50% of the patients who undergo a bone marrow transplantation will be alive 5 years later. Some groups of patients do have much better outcomes, such as patients with CML in first chronic phase undergoing a transplant from a sibling donor. On the other hand, older patients undergoing unrelated donor transplantation for acute leukemia in late remissions, such as second or third remission, might only have a 20% survival after 5 years. The reasons for an undesirable outcome are toxicity from the regimen, severe GVHD, or relapse of the underlying disease. Each of these three events occur for different reasons, and they vary between patients and the different diseases. It is best to discuss with your doctor what your odds are for your specific situation.

Bone Marrow Donor or Blood Stem Cell Donor

43. How long does it take to get a donor?

If your doctor recommends an allogeneic BMT for you, the choices of donor include siblings; other related donors, such as parents and children; and unrelated but matched donors. The process of HLA testing is relatively quick. After blood samples are obtained from the patient and potential donors, the determination of whether a match is available takes only 1 to 2 weeks. If a more extensive search for an unrelated donor must take place, the time required to identify and confirm a donor's eligibility takes up to several months. The initial process consists of a computer check for how many potential donors exist in the national registry. When potential donors are identified, further laboratory testing must be done on samples to determine whether the match is a full match or a partial match; this process can take 1 to 2 months. When a donor is identified, the individual must be cleared medically by his or her physician to be a stem cell donor. The stem cell donor is required to either have a **bone marrow harvest** under general anesthesia in the operating room or, increasingly, to have peripheral blood stem cells collected, in a process called **apheresis**.

Apheresis involves receiving a growth factor such as **granulocyte colony-stimulating factor** (G-CSF, a growth factor given to activate production of cells) by injection for several days, followed by the placement of

Bone marrow harvest

Under general anesthesia, marrow is collected for later infusion into the patient.

Apheresis

The process of having peripheral blood stem cells collected.

Granulocyte colony-stimulating factor

Growth factors given to activate production of cells.

an intravenous catheter to remove blood for the purpose of filtering the blood on a cell separation device.
The donor reclines in a collection chair while the
blood is removed and centrifuged to remove the fraction of cells that contain stem cells. This process takes
several hours daily for 1 to 3 days. The collection is
stopped when it is determined that sufficient stem
cells were obtained.

44. If I have an unrelated donor transplantation, do I get to meet the donor?

The current rules and regulations used by the National
Marrow Donor Program (NMDP) are that the identity
of an unrelated donor is confidential in the first year after
transplantation. After this, the identity of the donor can
be revealed. Frequently, attempts are made by the donor
and recipient to meet personally and share experiences
and celebrate. This can be a very emotional experience for
both the donor and the recipient, as well as their families.

45. Where do the donors come from?

National Marrow Donor Program

A large registry with millions of potential donors for future stem cell transplants.

The **National Marrow Donor Program (NMDP)** is
one of several large registries with several millions of
potential donors in its files. Donors have volunteered
to have their blood typed for the availability of a stem
cell transplant in the future. Many donors have come
forward during blood drives or answer the needs of a
particular patient or family member of whom they are
aware. Donors are literally everywhere in the world,
and the American NMDP registry can tap into international registries. In the United States, most donors
end up being selected from one of the over 4 million
registered donors in the NMDP. Hematopoietic stem
cells, bone marrow or blood, are collected at the site
where the donor has registered. The cells are flown to

the transplant center where the patient will undergo the transplantation. The process of infusing the donor stem cells into the hospitalized patient through an intravenous line takes from 1 to several hours. It is almost always uneventful, but minor (and reversible) allergic reactions can take place, similar to those in blood transfusions. The patient is always carefully observed during the stem cell infusion process, which may seem like a "non-event" after all the preparation, chemotherapy, and testing that has led up to this important time.

46. Is a sibling or family member always the best donor choice?

The answer is almost always "yes." However, **HLA-matched siblings** must be perfectly matched at the histocompatibility antigens currently tested. If the sibling is not matched for at least five of the six major antigens, then an alternative donor might be the best choice. Some transplantations are performed using children of the patient or a parent of the patient as the donor. Almost always, there is significant mismatching in this situation, but if only one or two antigens are mismatched, this may be the patient's best option. Although this is a less-than-optimal situation, many successful transplants have been performed in this manner.

HLA-matched sibling

Compatible sister or brother who is determined by testing to be matched at specific loci.

47. Is a young donor better than an older one?

This is a complicated question. In general, a young donor is probably superior to an older donor within some limits. Between the ages of 20 and 50, there is probably not that much difference between donors. It might be difficult to obtain stem cells from older donors in particular, such as those over 60. However, typically, if a donor is on the younger side, that would mean that the patient is probably on the younger side as well, given that the age range of most full siblings is usually not more than 15 to 20 years. And usually, the age range is much less; thus, a sibling donor is likely to be close to the same age as the patient. Thus, outcomes of such transplantations are much more related to the age of the patient than that of the donor.

48. Does my blood type change after BMT?

The red cell blood type changes to that of the donor after BMT. That means that if the patient has blood type A before transplantation and the donor is blood type O, eventually the patient will end up with blood type O. It may take several weeks to months for the "A" blood cells to totally disappear, but they eventually will. Occasionally, after transplantation in the situation just described, antibodies formed by the donor lymphocytes destroy the red blood cells of the recipient of type A. This can sometimes cause clinical problems, such as pain and rapid red blood cell destruction with severe anemia. Usually, however, the process is relatively silent and benign. The histocompatibility antigens (human leukocyte antigens, HLAs) of the blood cells also change after allogeneic transplantation. The donor cells will engraft, and all blood cells then take on the HLA identity of the donor.

Human leukocyte antigen (HLA)

The protein on the surface of all cells that must be matched for bone marrow transplants.

49. Can I still be an organ donor after transplantation? How about a blood donor?

A diagnosis of cancer excludes an individual from being either an organ donor or a blood donor. Therefore, even though the leukemia has been cured, the need for extreme caution in maintaining a safe blood supply as well as the need to "do no harm" to a potential organ recipient dictates that a former leukemia patient cannot donate his or her tissues to other patients.

PART FIVE

Side Effects and Complications of Treatment

Will I need blood transfusions?

More ...

50. Will I need blood transfusions?

Patients treated for leukemia often need to have **blood transfusions** as a consequence of the chemotherapy or because the disease itself has led to significant anemia or thrombocytopenia (low platelet count). Blood transfusions replenish red blood cells in the bloodstream when your own bone marrow is unable to do so. A threshold level of blood hematocrit or hemoglobin is selected by most physicians or hospitals for the use of blood transfusions to be considered (see Question 16). Because fatigue and shortness of breath are common symptoms of anemia, a blood transfusion usually makes the patient feel better almost immediately. Once it is determined that blood is needed, a unit of blood generally takes about 60 minutes to infuse into the patient. Generally, two units of blood are ordered, but occasionally, a physician may order only one unit to be infused.

Platelet transfusions
Procedures used in cancer patients to prevent or control bleeding when the number of platelets has decreased.

Platelet transfusions may be given if your platelet count reaches a critical level, as determined by your physician. Prophylactic platelet transfusions help prevent serious bleeding, a problem that can be life threatening when the platelet count is very low. Patients with acute leukemia generally need to undergo platelet transfusions during the intense phase of their treatment, and patients with chronic leukemia might need platelet transfusions in the later stages of their disease.

51. Are blood transfusions safe?

The simple answer to this question is "yes." Screening for blood donors is very rigorous in order to exclude the transmission of infectious agents. Patients with high-risk behaviors, such as intravenous drug use or unprotected sex, are not allowed to donate blood under any circumstances. All donor units are screened for human immunodeficiency virus (HIV) and hepatitis B and C viruses. With this kind of testing, the risk of acquiring the hepatitis C virus is less than 1 in 100,000 units, the risk of acquiring hepatitis B virus is less than 1 in 63,000 units, and the risk of acquiring HIV is less than 1 in 750,000 units.

There are other, noninfectious risks of blood transfusion, including sudden destruction of the transfused red cells or even late destruction of the transfused red cells. This can give rise to serious complications, including kidney failure. However, these are very rare, and the benefit of transfusion far outweighs this small risk. Some patients also have a slight fever after blood transfusion, which can be treated with acetaminophen (Tylenol).

Circulatory overload can occur occasionally in somebody with underlying congestive heart failure, but slow administration and perhaps the use of a diuretic medication can prevent this. Platelet transfusions carry the same infectious risks as blood transfusions, but they are equally well screened for infectious agents. Reaction to platelets sometimes occurs, consisting of fevers and chills. Again, this may be treated with medications like Tylenol. The decision to give a blood or platelet transfusion is taken very seriously by a physician. When the decision is made to transfuse blood or platelets, the physician has determined that the benefits to the patient far outweigh any risks.

Blood products to be transfused into patients with leukemia are filtered to remove white blood cells in order to decrease potential immunization to white blood cell antigens that may lead to the development of auto-antibodies; these auto-antibodies could, in turn, lead to destruction of platelets. In addition, blood and platelet units are treated with radiation to destroy white blood cells that might attack the patient (causing graft-versus-host disease; see Questions 63–65) while he or she is immunosuppressed by chemotherapy. Filtration and irradiation have made blood cell transfusions much safer, allowing the life-saving nature of these treatments to be employed widely for leukemia.

52. What side effects might a patient experience with chemotherapy?

Side effects

Usually describes situations that occur after treatments. For example, hair loss may be a side effect of chemotherapy; fatigue may be a side effect of radiation therapy.

Analgesic

Medicine given to control pain.

Mucositis

A temporary but painful condition in which the lining of the inside of the mouth breaks down, making eating and swallowing difficult.

The **side effects** that are most common with leukemia patients include stomach upset up to the level of nausea and vomiting, mucositis (sore mouth), osteoporosis (thin bones), muscle weakness, severe energy depletion, reduced mental awareness, loss of appetite, blurred vision, loss of sexual desire, and headaches. The immediate effects of chemotherapy, such as nausea and vomiting, can be very well controlled with anti-nausea medications, and **analgesics** are available to handle the worst of the pain. The worst side effect of chemotherapy is the reduction in your blood counts, leading to anemia, low platelet count, and low white blood cell count. Until chemotherapy or biologic therapy exists that can target only the leukemia cells, this side effect is unavoidable. **Mucositis** occurs when the lining of the inside of the mouth breaks down, making even swallowing painful. Liquid morphine is often prescribed for a short period so that patients can get adequate nourishment without experiencing the pain of mucositis. As the white counts continue to recover, this condition gradually abates.

All drugs are filtered through the body by the kidneys or are metabolized (broken down) by the liver. It is very important when you are taking these treatments that you constantly flush your body with fluids. When you are in the hospital, you are usually given an intravenous infusion of a saline solution for that purpose. You may experience a continuing urge to urinate—this is not always pleasant because being in bed and hooked to several intravenous lines makes it a real challenge to get up for relief. In this case, bedpans become essential. When you leave the hospital, you will be instructed to drink plenty of fluids, and this may continue until your drug therapy is discontinued, and kidney functions return to normal. You should have no alcoholic beverages until all medications are discontinued because alcohol inhibits the bone marrow, thus slowing down the recovery from chemotherapy. Alcohol may also injure your liver.

Drugs used to treat acute leukemia affect rapidly dividing cells. Unfortunately, hair follicles fall into that category. Therefore, it is fairly universal that patients with acute leukemia will lose their hair (**alopecia**) during chemotherapy. This means *all hair*. Remember that the hair will grow back. The loss of hair lasts for about 4–6 weeks, beginning about 7–14 days after the start of treatment. In some cases, the regrown hair will be slightly different in color and texture. That is only temporary, and the hair eventually will be the same as before (see Question 60).

Alopecia
Hair loss.

53. Will I lose weight after chemotherapy?

Typically, you will lose weight during treatment. When you are in the hospital, it will be harder to consume an adequate number of calories because of the nature of cafeteria-style food and the lack of appetite induced by chemotherapy. However, it is important to maintain your nourishment. If your physician and dietitian agree, indicate that you would like food brought in from home that meets their standards, but that would also taste good. You may find that much of the time, you have difficulty tolerating food due to mucositis and nausea. You may also notice a change in the way certain foods taste. This is only temporary, and taste returns to normal after the medications are discontinued.

54. Are there any proven herbal remedies that reduce side effects, or that have therapeutic effects?

Alternative medicine

Nontraditional medical supplements or techniques.

Antiemetic

Medicine that prevents or relieves nausea and vomiting, used during and sometimes after chemotherapy.

There is great interest in **alternative medicine** (i.e., nontraditional medical supplements or techniques) in the United States at this time. At the time of this writing, there are no known herbal remedies to reduce side effects. Modern antinausea drugs (called **antiemetics**), blood cell growth factors, and antibiotics are doing a great job in limiting side effects already. In addition, despite claims that mushroom extracts and other so-called natural remedies have therapeutic effects in leukemia and other cancers, there is no credible evidence to back up these assertions. *In fact, some products may even be harmful.* The patient should beware of information from the Internet and nonscientific publications that may give the impression that the cure for your leukemia is somehow being kept secret. Patients should not consider information regarding alternative medicines or treatments found in print or Internet advertisements to be credible and unbiased. The FDA must approve all medicines used in the United States, and investigational medicines must have FDA clearance for studies of their safety and efficacy. Currently, however, the FDA does not regulate dietary supplements, which is why some outrageous claims are allowed to go unchallenged. Feel free to discuss something you may have read with your doctor. He or she should be able to assure you that you are already receiving the best possible medicines and treatments and that you should not resort to unproven methods of treatment. If you are not convinced, perhaps you might seek a second opinion.

55. Do I need to be in the hospital to receive treatment?

It depends. Some leukemia treatments can easily be given in an outpatient setting. For example, oral drug therapy with Gleevec for CML is entirely an outpatient treatment. On the other hand, the treatment of acute leukemia with combination chemotherapy usually is administered intravenously and sometimes by long infusion and requires hospitalization. Modern practice usually involves discharging the patient after the chemotherapy itself has been administered. Readmission to hospital may be necessary for treatment of complications, such as infection or bleeding. The most common reason for readmission to the hospital is the treatment of systemic infection, the signs of which are usually fever and chills, fatigue, and a generally poor feeling (known as **malaise**).

Malaise

A condition marked by fatigue and overall poor feeling.

73

56. What types of infections do I need to be concerned about?

There are many infections that complicate treatment of leukemia or that are increased in frequency because of the leukemia itself. Patients with CML do not have a particularly high incidence of infection. Patients with CLL, on the other hand, do have a higher incidence of bacterial infections. If you have CLL and are receiving drug treatment, you would be at risk for pneumonia or other upper respiratory infection at a rate higher than the normal population.

Patients with acute leukemias are the most vulnerable to infections, and the risk depends on many factors, such as the level of neutrophils in the blood, how recently you had chemotherapy, and host factors, such as age and general medical condition. Bacterial infections are most common, followed by viral infections, followed by fungal infections. Fever is usually the first sign of infection that should be called to your doctor's attention. Of course, patients with leukemia can also get the common cold, upper respiratory infections, and the flu. It may be difficult to differentiate some conditions from a more serious bloodstream infection by a bacterium during neutropenia. Your doctor should be told of any new symptoms that are noticed, particularly when you are undergoing treatment, or if you are neutropenic.

57. Are all complications treatable?

The treatment of leukemia involves the use of strong cytotoxic drugs that do not always differentiate normal from malignant cells (see Question 20). Those complications are reversible or treatable in that the symptoms can be managed. Many cytotoxic drugs cause nausea and vomiting, but routine use of very strong antinausea drugs has reduced the severity of this problem. Infections are certainly treatable. However, some patients do develop overwhelming infections that do not respond adequately to therapy, so although the infections are treatable, the treatment is not always successful. The treatment of childhood leukemia may result in some cognitive (thought) impairment, and possibly some slowness in growth and development.

The alopecia that occurs in most patients who undergo chemotherapy is temporary but, unfortunately, it has no known treatment while it lasts.

58. Will I need to wear a mask? Will I be in isolation?

Infections that are commonly encountered are caused by microorganisms that already have colonized your body. Therefore, measures taken to reduce exposure to organisms carried by others are only part of the story. If you are going to receive chemotherapy for acute leukemia in the hospital, you will probably have a single room that is considered clean and safe from airborne organisms. You will probably not wear a mask in your room, but if you leave the unit you may be asked to wear a mask to minimize exposure to infections carried by others. However, masks themselves do little to prevent the spread of infection. Correct and frequent hand washing should be emphasized, and anyone who visits the patients and enters the room must wash correctly. Wash stations are located outside of most patient hospital rooms. Patients may need to frequently remind even hospital staff to wash before entering or performing procedures. You will not be isolated from visitors, but reasonable limitations on large numbers of visitors, and of visitors with any signs of infection, are recommended. Children who recently have been immunized with live viruses (e.g., polio) should be avoided.

59. Will I be able to eat regular foods?

If you are being treated for one of the chronic leukemias, most likely you can eat whatever you desire. On the other hand, if you are under treatment for acute leukemia, you will have periods of low white blood cell counts because of both the disease and its treatment. During this time, you will need to be on a "neutropenic diet," that is, a diet that does not contain foods that might transmit infectious agents, such as bacteria, fungi, and parasites (see Question 15). This means no fresh fruits and vegetables or sushi and other raw meats. Once your blood counts have recovered, you will be able to eat your regular foods again. As with any person, it makes sense to eat a balanced diet complete with adequate fiber. If you are suffering from any lingering nausea or symptoms of indigestion, you may wish to consult a dietician at your doctor's practice. Avoiding spicy, fatty, or acidic foods is generally a good idea.

The taste buds are affected by chemotherapy. Therefore, for some weeks to months, food may not taste the same or be as pleasant as usual. However, normal taste sensations should recover with time.

60. How long before my hair grows back?

Depending on the particular chemotherapy agents that are given, regrowth of hair begins several weeks after the last chemotherapy administration. It will take several months for your hair to grow out fully. Notably, the color and texture of your hair may change on its return. Unfortunately, no remedy for hair loss with certain chemotherapy drugs has been found. Some patients cut their hair short before starting treatment to minimize the effect of the hair loss and to create an interesting new look.

Women are generally comfortable with wigs, and some like scarves or other homemade headgear. Men may get various hats to help mask the baldness. Although some people make a "fashion statement" and choose to shave their heads, for others, the loss of hair is a daily visual reminder that they are undergoing cancer treatment. As such, it is a constant reminder of the loss they are experiencing. Especially for these patients, presenting an attractive visual look to friends and family is extremely important and makes them feel more "normal." Because patients are in control of very little during this process, attention to head gear, wigs, hats, and so on, and presenting an attractive exterior to those around them empowers these patients and enhances their self-esteem at a difficult time in their lives. Often, patients in the hospital bring several soft caps that can be worn to sleep in, which make them feel more "presentable" to the various caretakers nurses and visitors with whom they come in contact.

61. What complications can I expect from total body irradiation (TBI)?

Total body irradiation (TBI) is associated with some nausea and vomiting during its administration. Like any therapy that will have effects on the bone marrow, it reduces blood counts and causes immunosuppression. Late side effects of TBI include the development of cataracts, hypothyroidism, joint necrosis, and possibly an increased incidence of secondary cancers, such as skin cancers and brain cancer. Secondary cancers as complications of TBI are rare, however. Despite these complications, TBI is an important ingredient of the preparative regimen for allogeneic transplantation for acute and chronic myeloid leukemia.

62. What is graft–versus–host (GVHD) disease and how is it related to BMT?

Graft-versus-host disease (GVHD) is a complication of allogeneic stem cell transplantation in which the lymphocytes from the donor's stem cells recognize certain antigens on the recipient (patient) as foreign. Thus, the lymphocytes mount a reaction against the tissues of the patient, causing GVHD. The organs particularly affected are the skin, the liver, and the gastrointestinal tract.

63. What are the consequences of GVHD?

GVHD manifestations can range from mild to severe. Mild GVHD may consist only of a minor skin rash that responds to steroid therapy. This mild reaction actually is generally associated with a better outcome because there is some evidence that GVHD correlates with a graft-versus-leukemia effect. **Graft-versus-leukemia effect** means that the donor's lymphocytes attack the patient's leukemia cells directly and help in the eradication of the leukemia.

However, if GVHD is quite severe, more aggressive medical therapy must be initiated, which can lead to

Graft-versus-host disease

Complication in which the lymphocytes from a donor's stem cells recognize certain antigens on the recipient (patient) as foreign.

Graft-versus-leukemia effect

Occurs when the donor's lymphocytes attack the patient's leukemia cells directly and help in the eradication of the leukemia.

more complications. Moreover, aggressive forms of GVHD may not respond well to therapy and may eventually actually lead to death. If your physician recommends that you have aggressive therapy to combat GVHD, discuss the ramifications and duration of this therapy so that you understand its consequences.

64. What are the differences between acute and chronic GVHD?

Acute GVHD is defined as GVHD that develops in the first 100 days after transplantation. The organs involved, including the skin, liver, and gastrointestinal tract, are primarily affected, leading to skin rash, jaundice, and diarrhea. *Chronic GVHD* is more subtle and affects different organs. For example, the eyes or the mouth may become dry, there may be a rash inside the mouth, the skin may develop a thickening and tightening, and there may be chronic liver dysfunction.

65. What is CMV?

CMV stands for **cytomegalovirus**. This virus is similar to the herpes virus and can cause pneumonia, hepatitis, and gastrointestinal illness. CMV is a relatively common virus, and most people have already been exposed to it. However, it can reactivate during immunosuppression and lead to disease in immunocompromised patients. A blood test can detect early initiation of CMV reactivation. If detected, "pre-emptive" drug therapy with a drug called ganciclovir can be initiated. Alternatively, patients may be treated with

Cytomegalovirus

A virus, similar to herpes virus, that can cause pneumonia, hepatitis, and gastrointestinal illness.

ganciclovir prophylactically (preventatively), irrespective of the results of the blood test.

66. Can I get the stem cell donor's allergies?

This has been described as a rare event after transplantation. It is not considered to be a major factor in choosing a donor because usually there is only one suitable donor, and the benefit of the therapeutic effect of the transplantation far outweighs any plausible risk of contracting an allergy.

67. What are other complications of stem cell transplantation?

As with chemotherapy in general for leukemia, the main complications of high-dose chemotherapy used in stem cell transplantation are infection, bleeding, and isolated **toxicity** to organs such as the liver, heart, lungs, or kidneys (rare). Organ toxicity is the state in which the organ may cease to function or functions ineffectively. Heart failure can occur rarely. Lung fibrosis and hypersensitivity reactions can occur after certain drugs are used in the transplantation process. The liver may develop a condition known as **veno-occlusive disease** that can lead to liver failure in some patients. In some patients who receive the drug cyclophosphamide, there can be bleeding from the bladder wall, leading to bloody urine for a period of days to weeks. There may be skin changes, such as darkened patches of skin known as **hyperpigmentation**. There may be changes in the finger- and toenails, such as nail dropout or splintering.

Veno-occlusive disease

A sometimes fatal condition that can lead to liver failure; requires rapid medical intervention.

Hyperpigmentation

Darkened patches of skin.

68. Do I lose my sexual desire after stem cell transplantation?

Many leukemia patients lose their sexual desire during and after their diagnosis and/or during treatment. The uncertainty of the future is difficult for most couples to put aside. When one partner is facing such a health challenge, the focus changes in the relationship to survival and how best to accomplish it.

During active treatment, your body will need all of its energy to fight the side effects. Any particular organ damage or dysfunction, such as kidney failure, will further play a role in how long the recovery process will take. Some medications will also inhibit your physical ability to have sexual activity. Over time, measured in weeks to months, as you recover from therapy, your sexual desire and your ability to perform will improve and should return to your normal pattern.

PART SIX

Treatment Facilities and Healthcare Providers

Are doctors always right?

Is there a difference between an attending doctor and a fellow?

More ...

69. Are doctors always right?

That is an easy question. Absolutely not. The first thing about being a good patient is that you need to be your own best advocate, along with your caregiver. Read, read, and read more. Be active on the Internet to view sites of nationally recognized organizations. Talk with others with leukemia. Confer with several doctors other than your own hematologist/oncologist about any issues that concern you. You will soon find out that there may be little consensus on just about anything you ask. The patient has the final say about what he or she will do. Patients are almost always free to decline any procedure and leave any facility at any time. Of course, they do this at their own risk. Most doctors have never been patients, so they do not always understand what their patients are going through and what is needed. In years past, the word "doctor" projected a God-like image. You could unquestioningly put your life in his or her hands, and the outcome would not be a concern. With the ever-changing medical arena and the increasing demands on our medical system, this attitude is outmoded. It is important to never let a doctor or nurse intimidate you when you have a medical question or need—all questions are important. The physicians who are licensed in this nation are the world's best trained and most dedicated, and most can do incredible things with their skills, knowledge, and dedication. Although patients like to think that their doctors are the best, no doctor is perfect. The medical community may never fully understand how the entire human body functions. That is why they call it *practicing* medicine. Thus, it cannot be assumed that every doctor has the same information and is capable of making the best decisions regarding your treatment. If you feel that someone who is treating you is not performing well, leave him or her quickly. As a patient,

The patient has the final say about what he or she will do.

you must have confidence in nurses and technicians, as well as physicians, caregivers, and all others who care for you. Time is not always on your side. Do not be intimidated. It is your life is at stake.

During your treatment for leukemia, many issues arise, and the answers you receive should be questioned if you don't clearly understand them. A physician's time can be very limited because of the increased caseload that most carry. Occasionally, physicians are not as informative or forthcoming as they could be. All questions or concerns should be answered on a daily basis while the doctor is examining the patient, whether the patient is hospitalized or under care in the outpatient setting.

There are great doctors, good doctors, and not-so-good doctors. One gauge for determining whether you have a great doctor is whether he or she always spends the appropriate amount of time to explain all issues in layman's terms to the patient and the caregiver. The doctor should always ask this question before leaving, "Do you have any further questions?"

The patient should always strive to acquire the best medical care available—the choice of physician can be the most important factor in a quick and successful return to good health. Second opinions are often recommended, especially if the clinical situation is not straightforward, or if the proposed treatment is not standard.

70. Is there a difference between an attending doctor and a fellow?

If you are being treated in a hospital setting, it is likely that you will be exposed to many different professionals. The medical team will be led by an **attending**

Attending physician

A fully licensed and board-certified/eligible physician who is on the faculty of the institution or the medical staff.

Fellow

A licensed physician who is still in training.

physician. This term applies to a fully licensed and board-certified/eligible physician who is on the faculty of the institution or the medical staff. A **fellow** is a licensed physician who is still in training. A fellow in hematology/oncology will have already completed 3 years of internal medicine training and likely will have taken boards in that discipline already. The certification agency is referred to as The American Board of Internal Medicine. At the completion of 2–3 years of hematology/oncology training, the fellow is then eligible to sit for the hematology and oncology boards, also administered by The American Board of Internal Medicine. Therefore, a fellow is a highly trained individual already, who is now honing his or her skills in the more specific discipline of hematology/oncology. You may also encounter medical residents, depending on the institution. Medical residents and interns are physicians who have received their medical degree from a certified medical school. They are in training in internal medicine, which is the parent discipline for hematology/oncology. You may also encounter medical students, who are in their third or fourth year of medical school. They will be under close supervision by licensed and certified physicians.

71. Do all hospitals perform all treatments?

With technology advancing daily, all hospitals are not capable of performing the most advanced tests and procedures that a leukemia patient might need. In addition, small community hospitals are not staffed for and oriented to the level of intensity of care that a leukemia patient requires. For this reason, we would recommend that chemotherapy for acute leukemia be delivered in a hospital that is prepared for the complications that may arise. This may or may not be an academic health center or a large experienced community hospital. In our estimation, the hospital should have a track record of delivering such treatments to at least 20 patients per year. Hospitals affiliated with major cancer centers are most likely to be oriented to the treatment of leukemia patients. The National Cancer Institute, a branch of the National Institutes of Health, recognizes certain institutions as either Clinical or Comprehensive Cancer Centers through a peer-reviewed mechanism that ensures quality. You are more likely to receive up-to-date care and access to innovative clinical trials at institutions that have met the high standards of the National Cancer Institute. However, many non-National Cancer Institute–designated cancer centers, hospitals, and private clinics may offer excellent services, too.

If a patient's leukemia is not responding to the **standard protocol** or if the treatment is causing other medical issues, clinical trials may be available (see Question 29). Hospitals and cancer centers have access to different clinical trials. If your hematologist/oncologist recommends or informs you of studies that are available, be sure to investigate all options available. Your doctor may inform you only of the ones that his or her hospital is performing and may not be aware of all that is available. Remember that patients are their own best advocates and must ask questions, and it is the patient's responsibility and right to do so. The Internet can be a very useful tool in locating information in this area, and the National Cancer Institute has a web page listing current, NCI-approved clinical trials. See Question 100 and the Appendix for some of the most common and useful web sites.

Standard protocol

Treatment generally recognized by the medical community as the standard of care.

72. Is there an agency with survival statistics for different treatments and BMTs?

The best source of information for leukemia treatments, including bone marrow transplantation, are the Leukemia and Lymphoma Society of America, the National Marrow Donor Program (NMDP), the Multiple Myeloma Association, the Myelodysplastic Foundation, the International Bone Marrow Transplant Registry, and the American Society of Bone Marrow Transplantation. The American Society of Hematology and the American Society of Clinical Oncology have useful information, as does the American Cancer Society. Contact information for these organizations can be found in the Appendix.

73. How important is the nurse's role in my overall care and survival?

Nurses are in the third most important category of caregivers in the life of a patient being treated for leukemia. Only your oncologist and caregiver are more essential. Nurses perform their duties and care as instructed by the physician.

The nursing shortage in this country is growing, and there are not enough qualified nursing schools to educate the amount of students that are needed. Hospitals have had to lower the standard of care by using technicians for patient care. With leukemia patients, this is of particular concern, because the care they need is very critical. Doctors instruct by writing or speaking orders, but the nurses carry out the elements of care. Aides or medical assistants have only 2 years of medical training, which is much different than a 4-year nursing degree. These personnel are very helpful in your care, but they require supervision.

The patient should talk to his or her nurse, and ask questions. It is your right as a patient to advise the charge nurse if you feel that you have an incompetent or inattentive nurse, and you should ask that nurse to be replaced by another. Remember that your health is at stake. It is also important to have your caregiver (see Questions 74–82) with you when all blood products are given. Most states require that two nurses check all data with you before blood is infused. You will need to answer several questions, including date of birth and social security number, for verification.

Because of the nationwide shortage of critical care nurses that exists today, providing the best care possible for leukemia patients is a difficult balancing act. Many nursing shifts are now being staffed temporarily by licensed vocational nurses (LVNs) instead of Registered Nurses (RNs) due to the shortage. Nurses brought in on a temporary basis are called traveling nurses. They contract with a medical facility for a short period (usually about 13 weeks). Although they are qualified professionals, most are not familiar enough with the facility and the staff to be able to offer the best possible care.

With this in mind, the need for accurate observation and documentation by your caregiver becomes even more important to the successful outcome of your treatment. If the patient or the caregiver is dissatisfied with the quality of care, the charge nurse should be contacted immediately. If the problem is not resolved, the director of nursing and the attending physician should be notified. Although the nurse's position is very demanding, the margin for error is very limited and should not be tested.

74. What are the functions of a caregiver?

Caregiver

Acts for the benefit of a patient at the time of serious illness or disease, on the patient's behalf, and to assist the patient in making decisions and choices.

Caregivers are very important to the outcome of a serious illness or disease. Each is part cheerleader, administrator, counselor, secretary, nurse, and chauffeur. The patient, at times, may be totally dependent on others to stay alive.

The caregiver steps in for the benefit of another at the time of serious illness or disease. The patient might be mentally fatigued by what seems like a relentless amount of medical advice and alternatives to treatment or may be physically challenged by the treatment itself. It is the role of the caregiver to not only be there for emotional support but also to help the patient decipher all of the information given, so that the patient is able to then make the best choice. The caregiver should have a willing spirit to go the distance and more when needed. A caregiver can be a spouse, family member, or friend.

The stress and the emotional and physical limitations of losing your health to leukemia are most difficult. You are faced with a tremendous number of critical decisions that could and will affect the chances of your survival. The patient needs a competent support structure of caregivers who are able to discuss issues as they arise and make decisions as necessary. Medications, lab tests, and procedures should all be documented—depending on the medical staff to always have all your details at their fingertips is unrealistic.

75. What should you expect from the caregiver/patient relationship?

The most important part of this relationship is a mutual respect for one another that allows the patient to trust the person who is responsible for the patient's well-being. The patient and the caregiver will spend an incredible amount of time together and will forge a relationship like no other. Leukemia is often an emotional roller coaster for both the patient and the caregiver. Thus, the caregiver will need to learn as much as possible about the patient's disease or illness and become familiar with the plan for medical care. The caregiver should always be on alert to the patient's emotional status, because a positive attitude is essential for the patient's successful recovery. The caregiver must be honest, forthcoming with information, kind, caring, and loving. He or she must be a good listener and a friend, and most importantly, must have patience.

76. How important is the caregiver to my survival?

It is very difficult to go through aggressive treatment for leukemia, particularly during periods of intense chemotherapy. Doing this alone would be very difficult for anyone. Therefore, the caregiver is most important for helping patients go through the acute phases of treatment. In addition to helping with basic needs, including eating, personal hygiene, and elimination, the caregiver also is extremely important for giving emotional support.

77. Should the caregiver keep a patient chart?

During chemotherapy and radiation treatments, a patient's physical and emotional well-being are taxed severely. Doctors present procedures that require decisions coupled with statistics that can often determine a patient's survival. The patient is constantly dealing with numbers—for blood counts, drug side effects, urination and stool quantities, and about all other medical issues. This requires someone, in addition to the medical staff, to keep accurate records. Doctors are very busy and go on rounds to see patients every day, asking many questions. If the caregiver can give answers quickly and accurately, the medical staff may be more forthcoming with patient information. This means that the patient and the caregiver will have a better understanding of the current medical conditions.

Keeping a detailed record of lab values and treatments is useful also in navigating the complexity of the health care system. Because you might be under the care of more than one doctor, any one doctor, hospital, or clinic may not have access to some or all of your medical records. An organized summary of events, kept in a notebook, can be very useful during an office or hospital visit.

The caregiver and the family need to keep communication toward the patient in the most positive and loving manner possible. This is most important in successfully surviving the most difficult time of life. Without a great caregiver, chances of a successful outcome are greatly reduced. Patients without family should have trusted and willing friends fill this role.

Patient advocate

An individual who serves the needs of the patient, who may be empowered to act on his or her behalf.

78. Are caregivers needed in the hospital?

Yes, most definitely. The caregiver is the **patient's advocate** when a patient is unable to make decisions personally. The patient must focus on getting well and not be sidetracked on issues that are best left up to others. The caregiver should make decisions on when best to step in if critical medical care is not being performed at the highest level.

While in the hospital, it is also important to have your caregiver available most of the time. The medical staff cannot provide support to patients as well as the family does. When problems arise, it is very helpful for the patient to have the support of loved ones. Having someone to talk with and discuss the current issues is a huge benefit.

Caregivers should never leave the patient unattended for any length of time. There must be someone with them throughout their stay to watch, listen, record, and ask questions about what is going on. Basically, the caregiver is a monitor to ensure that everything that is supposed to occur actually happens. If there is a problem, it should be reported; this is not a time to be silent for fear of hurting someone's feelings.

Hospitalizations can be long and arduous, filled with long days and nights. The caregiver should get rest when possible and take breaks when others come to visit the patient. The conversations should be kept light and positive. Patients are sometimes unable to see past the walls in the room, so they can easily become depressed, bored, and filled with anxiety. Music is often therapeutic and can be encouraged if the patient enjoys listening to tapes or CDs.

The food prepared in the hospital is often quite bland and may not appeal to the patient whose taste buds have been altered due to the therapy being given. With the approval and knowledge of the physician and dietician, the caregiver may be allowed either to supplement or fully attend to the patient's wishes for the nourishment desired. It is often a real treat to have some special food items brought in. This must be done cautiously because leukemia patients are immunosuppressed and could become very ill or even die if they ingest food that their systems cannot handle. The caregiver should always get permission before bringing food that is prepared out of the hospital to a patient.

79. Do caregivers get any training?

Many medical institutions have classes and groups in caregiving. After treatment and in-home care, the caregiver needs to administer medications and communicate with the hospital staff on a regular basis. Knowing what to do and how to do it is essential to accelerate the healing process. The patient's main goals should be to follow all the doctor's orders and to get discharged home as soon as medically possible. The caregiver is essential in helping to achieve these goals.

80. Can and should family members be caregivers?

Your family is most important, with each member filling different needs. Caregiving can be more demanding for the provider than for the patient because the patient is often medicated. The love and support from family members is often the single most reason that patients have to do their very best to survive during the most difficult of times. Fighting leukemia and going through the regimens of treatments is not for wimps—it is tough. The thought of not seeing your family any longer produces a great motivation. The best medication is unable to create such a response.

81. How involved should family members be with the patient?

Family members should be involved with the patient in order to provide emotional support. However, it is also important for family members to respect the privacy and the need for rest and solitude that the patient may need from time to time. Family members may be helpful in being the patient's advocate to the healthcare system. During the acute phases of treatment, the patient may not be in the position to question or may feel reticent about complaining. It is important for the family to be aware of what is going on with the patient and to make sure that symptoms are brought to the attention of the patient's doctor.

82. What is the impact of family as caregivers?

The positive impact that the family brings to a patient is enormous. The love and support from family are often the single biggest reason patients strive to do their best during the most difficult times. Each family member can fill different needs and accomplish different tasks. It helps to have a different face with a new conversation to help keep the mood uplifting and fresh. No medications can mirror a response as great as the love of a family member or close friend.

The love and support from family are often the single biggest reason patients strive to do their best.

83. Are all medical facilities the same?

Many patients feel that the larger the medical facility is, the better it must be. Sometimes, this may be the case, but assumptions should not be made when the stakes are so high. Before any treatment is performed, patients should visit a minimum of three centers and interview the physicians responsible for the care that their illness requires. With medical care, ignorance is not bliss. The patient must become as knowledgeable as possible in a short period of time. Talking to experts in the care and treatment of their disease is essential in gaining that knowledge.

Although most large cancer centers receive the greatest portion of government and private funding, the performance of smaller institutions should not be overlooked. Many excellent physicians prefer to practice in smaller centers where the bureaucracy is less intrusive and thus more time can be dedicated to the patients.

One criterion that may be used in evaluating the best possible facility is whether the institution has substantial experience in treating all types of leukemia. This assurance means that the doctors and all the support staff are equally experienced and are likely to be familiar with your particular type of leukemia.

Before you make the final decision, you should talk with some of the nurses and determine the level of care available at the facility. If chaos is the order of the day, that is not the place to receive care. Common sense can be as good as facts and figures. Patients must feel comfortable that they will receive the best care possible to encourage the necessary level of trust.

84. How can the patient show their appreciation toward their medical staff?

The patient's medical staff is like any other dedicated group of people. Professional personnel like to be shown respect and appreciation. These professionals involved in your care have a very demanding job. Tokens of gratitude are well advised and can make a difference in the attitude that a patient receives. As with any relationship, you receive what you put into it. These medical support members must care for people when they are, many times, at their worst. With this type of environment, an act of kindness goes a long way.

One of the authors of this book has a first-hand knowledge of this issue. After a bout with acute respiratory distress syndrome, a CML transplant patient awoke after being in a drug-induced coma for 10 days. He was so weak that he had to learn how to walk again, and his arm could not even bring a spoon of soup to his mouth. He had lost 30 of his original 140 remaining pounds. The patient became aware of the care that had been given to him by the staff members during the ordeal. How could a patient adequately express his gratitude?

One particular nurse was still in charge of this patient's care after he arrived from the intensive care unit. Once the patient was strong enough to walk a few steps, one late morning, the nurse guided him to the shower and held him up, spun him around under the spray, and washed him as he turned. This nurse was a retired Tampa Bay football player. Because two weeks had passed without this now-realized luxury of being clean, it was a most appreciated gesture. The patient insisted in treating his nurse to a gourmet lunch in the hospital cafeteria. He and the nurse proceeded down three floors. The patient bounced from side to side in the wheel chair during transport to celebrate the diversion (this was against regulations because the patient was still confined to the room). They entered the dining room and ate like they never had eaten before. During the meal, the charge nurse tracked them down. The nurse was summoned to retrieve the patient immediately and return him to his room. After finishing dessert, they returned and the nurse's female supervisor scolded the 240-pound ex-linebacker male nurse. The patient, in turn, called the director of nursing about his situation, saying how thankful he was for this side trip that included a rare hot and edible meal. A few days later, the patient was able to send a pair of front row baseball tickets to the nurse at his home. The patient, of course, is a co-author of this book. How thankful he is for this and many other simple pleasures he experienced during his hospital stay while battling leukemia!

85. What is the employer's responsibility to their employees pertaining to leave of absence for treatment of leukemia?

An employee is entitled to 12 weeks of family leave of absence (FMLA). The employee's same job or a comparable position is guaranteed on his or her return during these 12 weeks. Also, the health insurance benefits are continued as if the employee was still working during this time period. In other words, if the employee was paying $200 per month for his or her health insurance coverage, then the employee will continue to pay the same amount to the employer, and the benefits will continue through this period. In California and several other states, the employee can apply for state disability benefits so that additional income can be awarded while the employee is unable to work.

If the employee is unable to return to work after 12 weeks, the employer can terminate employment. In fact, most companies have a standard policy that is applied when the 12 weeks of FMLA are exhausted. At this point, the employee is removed from the payroll and the separation papers are completed. The employee is eligible by law to apply for continuation of health coverage (mandated by the Consolidated Omnibus Budget Reconciliation Act of 1985 [COBRA]). Under COBRA, the employer can charge the employee the full cost of the group healthcare plan plus a 2% administrative fee. In other words, if the employee has been paying $200 and the employer was paying the remainder of $300, the employee at this point could be responsible for $500 plus an additional 2%.

This healthcare continuation coverage is still under the employer's group plan. If payment from the employee is not received within 30 days of the date established by the employer each period, whether it is monthly or quarterly, the employer can cancel the health coverage at that time. It is advisable to send the funds by certified mail or in person and get documented receipts because this coverage is vital to your continued care. In most cases, the COBRA coverage continues by law for

18 months. If another qualifying event (e.g., death of a covered spouse) occurs, then the coverage extends to 36 months. A disability provision could extend the 18-month COBRA period to total coverage of 29 months. Because these issues can get rather complicated, and the laws can and do change, a good source of up-to-date information may be obtained from your local or state Chamber of Commerce.

86. When all else fails, how do I prepare my family and myself for my death?

Too few people think ahead to what happens should cancer get the better of them. Even knowing that leukemia can be a fatal disease, most people with it prefer to concentrate instead on curing the cancer—an understandable attitude that is to be encouraged. As time passes and the cancer advances, however, there comes a point when cancer patients should start thinking about what they want to have happen should they lose the battle. As difficult as it might be to contemplate your own death, doing so before the end is imminent can ease matters for you and your family if your leukemia follows that course. Everyone hopes to not need such arrangements any time soon, but it is useful to work out those legal arrangements that may be required ahead of time (while you're still feeling relatively good). Then, with the details of wills, power of attorney designation, do not resuscitate (DNR) orders (see Question 87), funeral arrangements, and other practical matters out of the way, it is easier to focus on your health, knowing that these structures are in place if necessary. There are several steps you can take to accomplish this.

It is useful to work out legal arrangements ahead of time.

Work toward acceptance. Even after a long, difficult illness, it's very hard to accept that you're going to die within the next few months or weeks. Preparing yourself for death is a major emotional and spiritual undertaking, so get assistance from a minister, social worker, or psychologist. If you don't have a minister or counselor with whom you're comfortable, most cancer centers or oncology wards have a chaplain or counselor in residence. Take advantage of their services, or ask for a referral. Involve your family in some of these sessions, but reserve as many as you need for yourself—if you can gain a sense of peace for yourself, it will help your family to cope with your death too. Ironically, achieving this sort of peace and acceptance can help you to live longer than predicted; it's not unknown for people who are believed to have but a few months remaining to live many months, even years, after making their "final" arrangements for death. You have a right to receive **palliative treatment**, a type of therapy that relieves symptoms, such as pain or fatigue, but does not alter the development of the disease. Its primary purpose is to improve the quality of a patient's life.

Because many people find this time hard to think about and talk about, it's likely that you'll have to raise the issue with your family, friends, and healthcare team. Your loved ones may resist the discussion, but be persistent—or get help from a social worker, counselor, or clergy who can guide them through this painful conversation. It's important to talk about what you want to happen in the final phases of your illness. Discuss the organization of personal documents and where they are kept so that your family and friends know what your wishes and desires are. Lawyers,

Palliative treatment

Therapy that relieves symptoms but does not alter the development of the disease. Its primary purpose is to improve the quality of life.

It's important to talk about what you want to happen.

clergy, and counselors may also help you and your family in planning for end-of-life issues.

Decide on the best place for your care. People facing advanced cancer should choose the location of their care: in the home, in an outpatient setting or the doctor's office, in the hospital, or through a hospice. Although a person can live with recurrent disease for a long time, at some point people with advanced disease experience a shift where it becomes clear that they are dying. It may be best to discuss the decision of where you would like to be treated for advanced cancer before this point if you can. Hospice care focuses on improving the quality of life for the remainder of your life and can make the process of dying as comfortable and as pain-free as possible. Hospice care can be given in the home, at the hospital, or in a separate hospice. These are all personal choices based on your needs and available resources. Your healthcare team can discuss these options with you and help you get the care you need.

Make your wishes known. If cancer treatment becomes unbearable, you have the right to request that your doctors stop treatment. You even have the ability to describe in writing what kinds of treatment you will and will not accept from them, in case you should lose the ability to communicate your wishes directly. Legal documents called **advance directives,** including living wills, durable power of attorney, DNR orders (see Question 87), and healthcare proxies, allow people to express their decisions regarding what they do and don't want to have done during their last weeks or months, in

Advance directives

Legal documents spelling out how you want your treatment to proceed, including living wills, DNR orders, and durable power of attorney.

case they become unable to communicate effectively at that time. These are described in Question 87.

87. Are there legal steps I can take to make my wishes known in case I'm not able to speak for myself near the end?

You have the right to decide what treatment you will and will not accept near the end of your life, and you also have the right to designate an individual to speak for you—this is usually a member of your family, but it can be a friend or an attorney. You don't need an official document or form—you don't even need to have this document written by an attorney. All you really need to do is sign a letter in the presence of two or more witnesses (who should also sign and date the document). However, if the letter is notarized, it will carry more weight with a hospital board, if questions should arise.

Advance directives dictate how you want your treatment to proceed, including living wills, DNR orders, durable power of attorney, and healthcare proxies. A **living will** simply outlines what care you want in the event that you become unable to communicate due to coma or heavy sedation. You're not locked into anything you write down. The document is nothing more than a legally valid guide for families and physicians to know a patient's thinking on how he or she should be cared for. If you change your mind about any of it, you can change the directives or even verbally countermand them to the physician treating you. Alternatively, you can limit the instructions to a **Do Not Resuscitate order (DNR)** if you decide differently, telling the medical staff at the hospital that they

Living will

Document outlining what care you want in the event that you become unable to communicate due to coma or heavy sedation.

Do Not Resuscitate order

A medical order telling the medical staff at the hospital or facility that they should not act to revive you in the event that your heart or brain activity cease.

should not act to revive you in the event your heart or respiratory activity (breathing) cease.

Even if you don't write it down, if you have certain ideas as to what kind of treatment you do and don't want, all you need to do is tell members of your family, particularly those acting as your principal caregivers. If they know your wishes, they can intervene on your behalf even without a written statement—although they may have to convince a judge that this is truly your wish, should the hospital balk at their requests to withhold treatment. Your family will then be bolstered if you prepare, in advance, a **durable power of attorney** (which allows a specific family member to legally make all your decisions, personal and financial, for you in case you become incapacitated). Another document you can prepare is a **healthcare proxy**, which limits the decision-making power to only those decisions regarding your medical treatment.

If you don't have a will, one should be written as soon as possible, particularly if you have children. If you fail to do this, most states' laws arrange for your assets to go directly to your spouse and children in specific proportions. However, processing your estate may take considerably more time without a will, which can cause problems for your family if bank accounts, property, or savings are held solely in your name. Different circumstances might create other mitigating factors—prior marriages with or without children, common-law marriages, or other nontraditional relationships. In these instances, having a will clarifies your wishes and is a tremendous kindness to your loved ones. Some people also make advance arrangements for their funerals, which can be particularly helpful to your family,

Durable power of attorney

Allows a specific family member to legally make all your decisions, personal and financial, for you in case you become incapacitated.

Healthcare proxy

Document that limits the decision-making power to only those decisions about your medical treatment.

because they won't be confronted with these details in the midst of grieving over your death. It might be difficult—there is no more stark confrontation with your impending mortality than arranging your own funeral. However, knowing that this detail is already dealt with can also help bring a measure of acceptance and peace.

PART SEVEN

Living with Leukemia

How do you know whether you are cured?

Will my child with leukemia grow up normally?

Do patients ever get back to normal?

More ...

88. How do you know whether you are cured?

Certain forms of leukemia are indeed curable. These include ALL, AML, and CML. Unfortunately, present treatments are generally not considered curative for CLL, although allogeneic bone marrow transplantation may cure some patients with this disease. Long-term follow-up of patients with acute leukemias and CML patients who have undergone allogeneic bone marrow transplantation have indicated that some patients never have a relapse. When sufficient follow-up has taken place over a number of years, it can be concluded that the patient is in fact cured. The first step toward cure is the achievement of a complete remission (total absence of disease) after initial therapy. In some cases, this may be determined by a examining the blood and bone marrow cells under a microscope to discover whether there are residual blasts. More refined techniques, such as molecular markers and chromosomal abnormalities, may be used as well to ensure that no hidden cells exist. There are certain prognostic features that predict with some certainty who is most likely to suffer a relapse; these are discussed in the section on cytogenetics (Question 18). In the initial phases of the remission, it is difficult to state with any certainty that a given patient is cured, because it takes a long follow-up to be sure that a cure really occurred. Thus, it is not easy for the physician to tell a patient that he or she is cured early after treatment. In the case of the acute leukemias after initial chemotherapy is completed, if the patient remains in complete remission for several years, it becomes more likely that the patient is in fact cured. Five-year survival numbers are often given when reporting outcomes of certain studies. Generally, if the patient survives 5 years after therapy, relapse is unlikely, but, unfortunately, not unheard of. Thus, the word "cure" must be taken with a grain of salt because a patient occasionally will relapse 7, 8, or more years after treatment.

Nonetheless, when a patient has survived for a long period of time after treatment, although there is some possibility of relapse, it becomes less common, and most patients have no difficulty putting their illness behind them. The fact that relapses can occur just means that the patient must continue to be followed up by his or her doctor.

CML is curable by allogeneic bone marrow transplantation. When performed in the first chronic phase, especially early after diagnosis of CML, allogeneic bone marrow transplantation has a very high cure rate, and the relapse rate is very low. If the transplantation is performed at a later stage of the disease, such as after a relapse, there is a higher probability of relapse. The new treatment recently established for CML using the drug known as Gleevec produces remissions in a large percentage of patients. At present, it is unknown whether these remissions will result in cures.

89. Will my child with leukemia grow up normally?

The combination of chemotherapy and central nervous system radiation therapy involved in the treatment of ALL does have a cost in terms of growth and development and neurologic function later in life. These effects are variable and seem to be more common in younger children (less than 5 years of age), and possibly more in girls than in boys. Survivors of childhood

ALL tend to have shorter height than their unaffected counterparts. There is also a higher incidence of cataracts and cardiac abnormalities. Gonadal function usually develops normally unless the patient has had prophylactic gonadal irradiation. Successfully treated children with ALL have gone on to bear normal children in adulthood. Secondary cancers, including brain tumors, acute myeloid leukemia, and rare carcinomas of the parotid and thyroid glands, are more common after treatment of ALL. Hopefully, new advances in treatment will allow less intense treatment or treatment with different agents that may decrease some of the side effects of treating ALL.

90. Do patients ever get back to normal?

In contrast to childhood ALL, patients treated for adult forms of leukemia who are successfully induced into remission will eventually find that they feel well and "normal" again. The time it takes to achieve this goal varies between patients and is affected by age and other medical illnesses or disorders that the patient may have. Lingering fatigue may plague a patient for several months or even a year, but it eventually improves, depending on the intensity of treatment that you achieved, any other illnesses you may have, age, prior fitness, and many other individual factors. Patients treated for the chronic leukemias may find that they feel much better after treatment has started because they may have with better blood counts and better control of side effects of the elevated white blood cell counts. Being treated with an agent like Gleevec, for example, is not really associated with very many side effects at all.

Lingering fatigue may plague a patient for several months or even a year, but it eventually improves

91. Do patients with leukemia develop other forms of cancer?

As mentioned earlier, children treated for ALL have a higher incidence of secondary neoplasms (cancers that develop later). Patients with CLL have a higher incidence of colon cancer and certain skin cancers. Patients treated for AML tend not to have a higher incidence of other cancers, if they are cured of the AML. Patients with CML do not have an increased incidence of secondary cancers. CML can evolve into a more aggressive form of leukemia that behaves essentially like AML.

92. Will I be able to have children?

Chemotherapy and radiation therapy can cause sterility. However, many patients who have been treated as children for acute leukemia have been able to have children of their own. For a young adult man, it would be advisable to collect sperm before chemotherapy or before bone marrow transplantation to ensure that he could later father a child through artificial insemination if he proves infertile. For women, it is possible to harvest and store ova (eggs), but the procedure is more invasive, and more expensive. In weighing the decision to collect sperm or harvest ova before treatment, bear in mind that fertility is still possible even after aggressive chemotherapy for adult leukemia. Nevertheless, many male and female patients do become sterile, and you must be prepared for this possibility.

93. When can I go back to work?

The answer to this question depends on the type of treatment you have received. Again, chronic leukemias may not necessitate ever leaving work unless the leukemia has advanced to an acute form or you undergo stem cell transplantation. Patients treated for acute leukemias need to stop working for some or all of the time during treatment. After the treatment has completed, the patient may resume work within a few weeks to months. If blood counts are depressed or there is ongoing immunosuppression, common sense approaches to avoiding infections will be recommended, such as avoiding crowds and washing frequently.

94. What are the patient's physical limitations after a bone marrow transplantation?

After an autologous transplantation, a patient usually bounces back to normal within a few months—there should really be no physical limitations. After an allogeneic transplantation, there may be numerous ongoing concerns, including active GVHD or active immunosuppression. The patient's blood counts and overall status generally dictate physical limitations. Certainly, walking and activities of normal daily living would be expected to return to normal within a few months, but vigorous exercise or exertion might not be recommended for several months to a year after transplantation (see Question 95).

95. When can a patient start to exercise after transplantation? Does exercise play a role in my recovery?

Light exercise—that is, walking and passive muscle movement—is recommended even during a bone marrow transplantation or chemotherapy in general. After completion of treatment, you should try to resume activities including walking and light exercise. If you have not been involved in vigorous exercise, this is probably not the time to start. However, if you have previously been physically fit and very involved in exercise routines, it is not unreasonable to gradually reintroduce your previous activities, depending on your blood counts and other physical factors. If anemia has been corrected and if low platelet counts are not a problem, then there are no true limitations to physical activities.

The general rule for exercise is a 20-minute routine a minimum of 3 days a week. This could be a brisk walk and some weight-bearing exercises, and can be done any time, your blood counts permitting and with your physician's permission. Everything should be done in moderation. The body will not perform at peak levels while in treatment. In many patients, this is frustrating. The key is to keep a routine going, especially if you are restricted to a bed for much of the day. During your treatment in the hospital, your doctor will encourage you to walk the halls regularly. In the first weeks, this will be very difficult. Exercise is good for patients physically and mentally to reduce anxiety and stress. The caregiver should help the patient stay motivated. You should consider consulting a physical therapist to give you instruction and ideas if routine exercise has not been a part of your daily life previously.

96. What is the chance of the leukemia coming back?

This question must be answered in relation to each form of leukemia as well as each stage and subtype of leukemia. This question also assumes that a remission has been achieved. If a patient with AML achieves a complete remission, then there is roughly a 60% chance that the disease will come back. If a child with ALL achieves a complete remission, the chance of recurrence is more like 20%. If an adult with ALL achieves complete remission, the chance of relapse is more like 60%. Patients with CML are currently being treated with the new drug, Gleevec. At this time, it is uncertain what the relapse rate will be in those who do respond to the drug. Patients with CLL generally cannot achieve remission with current available therapies. After bone marrow transplantations, the relapse rates are also variable, depending on the disease and when the transplantation was performed. For example, if the patient has AML and undergoes an autologous transplantation in first complete remission, the relapse rate is approximately 40%. If the patient undergoes an autologous transplantation in second complete remission, the relapse rate is 60%. If a patient with CML undergoes an allogeneic stem cell transplantation, the relapse rate is approximately 10% in chronic phase, 30% in accelerated phase, and 50% in blastic crisis. Thus, the overall complexity of the variables involved in the leukemia, its biology, the mode of treatment, and other factors all influence the relapse rate, and it is best to discuss these with your doctor to get a more precise probability.

97. What should I do about routine immunizations? Should I still get a flu shot every year?

After treatment for leukemia with standard chemotherapy, it is not necessary to be re-immunized for childhood illnesses. Of course, you still need to keep up with your tetanus shots, which should be given every 10 years, and an annual flu shot is recommended for adults. In addition, the pneumonia vaccine should be given every 3 years. Special considerations exist for patients who undergo blood or marrow stem cell transplantation. *Re-immunization against tetanus, mumps, hepatitis B, and pneumococcal pneumonia may be recommended after you are off immunosuppressive drugs.*

98. What are your legal rights as an employee undergoing treatment?

Like most other serious illnesses, leukemia alters your ability to perform your job. If you are employed, it is wise to seek counsel on what legal protections are available to you in your state. Most states have laws in place that extend your medical insurance for an additional length of time. It is critical for the employee to keep in contact with the human resources department at your job to be sure that the medical insurance premiums are paid and there is no lapse in coverage.

Most employers are sympathetic to the seriousness of the situation. Knowing the amount of time you are likely to be off, and the laws of the state in which you reside, it is wise to be as candid about the situation as is reasonably possible. In this way, your employer will realize that you are sincere and trustworthy about the information that you are revealing. Employers do not want to lose good employees. It is in their best interest to do all that is necessary to help you win this fight. Depending on what type of job you have and what your treatment is, it is not uncommon to be off the job from several months to more than a year. If your position is physical or requires public contact, then this will be more difficult. Some patients with office or

It is not uncommon to be off the job from several months to more than a year.

sales positions can telecommute, which is desirable because much of the recovery is slow and boring, but not always that taxing.

99. What about the cost and insurance coverage for treatment?

Anyone with leukemia will need to spend time communicating with his or her insurance carrier, because the medical costs are significant and can be catastrophic if not handled well. In most cases, the hospital or physician's office is the mediator with the insurance company as they seek authorization for the proposed treatment plan. Insurance companies almost always consider leukemia a covered illness, but the treatments they cover may not be fully paid. There also may be differences between payment of outpatient versus inpatient treatments. If you have health maintenance organization coverage, it is wise to keep the treatment within network facilities, because treatment there is usually covered at a higher percentage than at out-of-network facilities. Contact your insurance company or ask a patient representative at your doctor's office to determine what coverage is available.

Explanation of benefits

A statement of covered assessments and treatments that is provided by the insurance carrier.

The insurance carrier will send you an **explanation of benefits (EOBs)**. These statements explain the amount of the invoice, what the contract price is, and what they will pay. Most of the time, they also advise you about what your financial obligation will be. Do NOT pay any invoices that are covered by insurance without first receiving your copy of the EOB. It is estimated that up to 80% of medical invoices charged to patients have errors. Your caregiver should monitor all procedures and document them for you.

100. Where can I get more information about leukemia?

The information in this book just scratches the surface of what's available to leukemia patients and their families. The accompanying appendix offers a selection of good resources to address many topics. Numerous pamphlets and handouts are also provided by medical institutions so that potential patients can discuss all options available. Be sure to ask for these handouts and any others as they become available. The outpatient clinic where patients are receiving treatment is a good source for up-to-date information via flyers, posters, and handouts.

Many web sites contain information helpful to patients and physicians. One of the most relevant is that of the Leukemia and Lymphoma Society of America (web site: *www.leukemia-lymphoma.org*). The International Bone Marrow Transplant Registry (IBMTR) (web site: *www.ibmtr.org*) posts summary results of hematopoietic stem cell transplantation listed by diseases and **staging** (the extent of the disease), as well as results of autologous versus allogeneic transplantation. The National Marrow Donor Program (NMDP) (web site: *www.marrow.org*) lists the requirements of becoming a hematopoietic stem cell donor and information for potential donors. The American Society of Hematology (ASH) (web site: *www.hematology.org*) is another organization that has helpful education material. The American Association of Blood Banks (AABB) (web

Staging

Evaluating the extent of the disease.

site: *www.aabb.org*) provides information about becoming a blood component donor and current tests that are performed on each unit of blood to minimize diseases associated with transfusion. The Foundation for the Accreditation of Hematopoietic Cell Therapy (FAHCT) (web site: *www.fahct.org*) is a organization that produces standards for hematopoietic stem cell transplantation, inspects transplantation centers, and accredits those programs that have met their stringent criteria. The National Leukemia Research Associations (also called the National Leukemia Research Association) has a web site that appears to address only children's illnesses, yet information on adult leukemia is presented here as well because their web site has expanded (*www.childrensleukemia.org*). Many nurses belong to the Oncology Nursing Society, whose web site is *www.ons.org*. Information about other considerations is found at The Wellness Community's web site at *www.cancer-support.org*. Spouses seeking support and information can review material at *www.wellspouse.org*, operated by the Well Spouse national organization.

Other academic societies and organizations associated with leukemia that frequently post important and relevant information in their web sites include the American Society of Clinical Oncology (ASCO) (web site: *www.asco.org*) and the International Society for Experimental Hematology (ISEH) (web site: *www.iseh.org*). In addition, you may wish to visit the web site of your local healthcare providers, such as major hospitals and cancer centers.

Appendix

American Cancer Society
1599 Clifton Road
Atlanta, GA 30329
Phone: 800-ACS–2345
Web site: *www.cancer.org*

Blood and Marrow Transplant Information Network
2900 Skokie Valley Rd, Suite B
Highland Park, IL 60035
Phone: 888–597–7674 or 847–433–3313
Web site: *www.bmtinfonet.org*

The Bone Marrow Foundation
70 East 55th Street, 20th floor
New York, NY 10022
Phone: 800–365–1336
www.bonemarrow.org

Cure for Lymphoma Foundation
215 Lexington Ave, 11th Floor
New York, NY 10016
Phone: 800–235–6848 or 212 213–9595
www.cfl.org

International Bone Marrow Transplant Registry (IBMTR)
Medical College of Wisconsin
P.O. Box 26509
Milwaukee, WI 53226
Phone: 414–456–8325
www.ibmtr.org

Leukemia & Lymphoma Society of America
Phone: 800–955–4572
for local chapter information
www.leukemia-lymphoma.org

National Cancer Institute (NCI)
Cancer Information Service
Bldg. 31, Room 10A07]
900 Rockville Pike
Bethesda, MD 20892
Phone: 800–422–6237
www.nci.nih.gov

National Leukemia Research Associations
AKA National Leukemia Research Assn.
585 Stewart Avenue
Suite 18
Garden City, NY 11530
Phone: 516–222–1944
Fax: 516–222–0457
www.childrensleukemia.org

NOTE: while it states only "children's leukemia", there is
information on adult leukemia too.

National Marrow Donor Program (NMDP)
3001 Broadway Street NE, Suite 500
Minneapolis, MN 55413
Phone: 800–654–1247 or 612–627–5800
Office of Patient Advocacy
Phone: 888–999–6743
www.marrow.org

Oncology Nursing Society
501 Holiday Drive
Pittsburgh, PA 15220
Phone: 412–921–7373
www.ons.org

The Wellness Community
8044 Montgomery Road, Suite 170
Cincinnati, OH 45236
Phone: 888–793-WELL
www.cancer-support.org

Well Spouse Foundation
30 E. 40th Street
New York, NY 10016
Phone: 800–838–0879 or 212–685–8815
www.wellspouse.org

Acute: Occurring suddenly in a short period of time.

Acute lymphocytic leukemia: Rapidly growing leukemia affecting mature lymphocytes.

Acute myeloid leukemia: Rapidly growing leukemia affecting mature white cells.

Advance directives: Legal documents spelling out how you want your treatment to proceed, including living wills, DNR orders, and durable power of attorney.

ALL: See acute lymphocytic leukemia.

Allogeneic bone marrow transplantation: Bone marrow transplantation using marrow from another person's body.

Allogeneic stem cell transplantation: Cells from another's body are used to treat a cancer.

All-*trans*-retinoic acid: A drug related to vitamin A that is able to make certain leukemia cells change from blasts to normal mature cells.

Alopecia: Hair loss.

Alternative medicine: Nontraditional medical supplements or techniques.

AML: See acute myeloid leukemia.

Analgesic: Medicine given to control pain.

Anesthesia: Medication that causes entire or partial loss of feeling or sensation.

Antibody: Any of the body's immunoglobulins that are produced in response to specific antigens.

Antiemetic: Medicine that prevents or relieves nausea and vomiting, used during and sometimes after chemotherapy.

Antigen: Substance capable of stimulating an immune response.

Anti-sense therapy: Emerging investigational therapy for various diseases that blocks protein production.

Apheresis: The process of having peripheral blood stem cells collected.

Aspirate: Removing fluid or cells from tissue by inserting a needle and drawing the fluid into the syringe.

Asymptomatic: Without obvious signs or symptoms of disease.

Attending physician: A fully licensed and board-certified/eligible physician who is on the faculty of the institution or the medical staff.

ATRA: See all-*trans*-retinoic acid.

Atypical cells: Not usual; abnormal. Cancer is the result of atypical cell division.

Autoimmune process: A reaction of a person's immune system against tissues in his or her own body.

Autologous: Coming from the same person.

Autologous stem cell transplantation: Cells from the patient's own body are used to treat cancer.

Biopsy: Surgical removal of a small piece of tissue or a small tumor for microscopic examination to determine whether cancer cells are present. A biopsy is the most important procedure in diagnosing cancer.

Blast: An immature white blood cell that normally represents an early phase of the normal differentiation process that occurs in the bone marrow.

Blood count: A test to measure the number of red blood cells, white blood cells, and platelets in a blood sample.

Blood transfusion: Replenishment of red blood cells in the bloodstream when one's own bone marrow is unable to do so.

Bone marrow: The soft, fatty substance filling the cavities of the bones. Blood cells are made here.

Bone marrow biopsy and aspiration: A procedure in which a needle is inserted into the center of a bone, usually the hip, to remove a small amount of bone marrow for microscopic examination.

Bone marrow harvest: Under general anesthesia, marrow is collected for later infusion into the patient.

Bone marrow transplant: A procedure in which the bone marrow of a leukemia patient is replaced by another person's marrow.

Cancer: A general term that describes over 100 different uncontrolled growths of abnormal cells in the body. Cancer cells have the ability to continue to grow, invade and destroy surrounding tissue.

Cancer cell: A cell that divides and reproduces abnormally with uncontrolled growth. If this cell breaks away and travels to other parts of the body, it is referred to as metastasis.

Carcinogen: Any substance that initiates or promotes the development of cancer.

Caregiver: Acts for the benefit of a patient at the time of serious illness or disease, on the patient's behalf, and assists the patient in making decisions and choices.

Catheter, indwelling: Device placed surgically beneath the skin to facilitate the frequent infusion of medications and/or other treatments (see Port-A-Cath).

CBC: See complete blood count.

Cell: The basic structural unit of all life. All living matter is composed of cells.

Chemotherapy: Treatment of cancer by use of chemicals; often uses two or more chemicals to achieve maximum kill of tumor cells. Usually refers to drugs used to treat cancer.

Chronic lymphocytic leukemia: A slow-growing leukemia that affects mature lymphocytes.

Chronic: Occurring more slowly and present less dramatically than acute conditions.

Chronic myeloid leukemia: A slow-growing leukemia of mature white blood cells, associated with the Philadelphia chromosome.

Clinical trial: A specific treatment protocol that is designed to test the effectiveness and safety of a drug or combination of drugs, or other therapies, in the treatment of a disease.

Chromosomes: Large complex structures that contain DNA and proteins.

CLL: See chronic lymphocytic leukemia.

CML: See chronic myeloid leukemia.

CMV: See cytomegalovirus.

COBRA: Consolidated Omnibus Budget Reconciliation Act of 1985; ensures continuation of health coverage offered by insurance companies.

Complete blood count: A laboratory test to determine the number of red blood cells, white blood cells, platelets, hemoglobin and other components of a blood sample.

Complete remission: Total absence of disease.

Congenital disease: A disease existing at or dating from birth.

Consolidation: Additional chemotherapy after remission, often given in cycles.

Cytogenetic analysis: A procedure whereby cells, taken from either the blood or the bone marrow, are cultured in a specialized laboratory in such a way that the dividing cells are arrested in the middle of their division. The structure of the chromosomes can then be stained and visualized by a microscope.

Cytomegalovirus: A virus similar to herpes virus, which can cause pneumonia, hepatitis, and gastrointestinal illness.

Cytopenia: Low blood count.

Cytotoxic: Drugs that can kill cancer cells. Usually refers to drugs used in chemotherapy treatments.

Differentiation: The process during which the stem cell goes through several stages of development.

Diagnosis: The process of identifying a disease by its characteristic signs, symptoms, and laboratory findings.

DNA: One of two nucleic acids (the other is RNA) found in the nucleus of all cells. DNA contains genetic information on cell growth, division, and cell function.

DNA-damaging agents: Known to be initiators of leukemia, including chemicals (benzene and other solvents), ionizing radiation, and some other organic compounds.

DNR order: See Do Not Resuscitate order.

Donor: One who donates blood stem cells or bone marrow for infusion into a patient.

Do Not Resuscitate order: A medical order telling the medical staff at the hospital or facility that they should not act to revive you in the event that your heart or brain activity cease.

Durable power of attorney: Allows a specific family member to legally make all your decisions, personal and financial, for you in case you become incapacitated.

EOB: See explanation of benefits.

Explanation of benefits: A statement of covered assessments and treatments that is provided by the insurance carrier.

Flow cytometry: A test performed on cancerous tissues that shows the aggressiveness of the tumor.

FDA: See Food and Drug Administration.

Fellow: A licensed physician who is still in training.

FMLA: See family leave of absence

Food and Drug Administration: A federal institution charged with approving and regulating medications, foodstuff, and other products for human consumption.

Genes: Located in the nucleus of the cell, genes contain hereditary information that is transferred from cell to cell.

Gene therapy: Investigational treatment of disease by the introduction of new genetic material into cells in order to modify their DNA.

Genetic: Refers to the inherited pattern located in genes for certain characteristics.

Gleevec: Oral chemotherapy agent approved for use in patients with CML.

GVHD: See graft-versus-host disease.

Granulocyte: White blood cell with a large number of granules.

Graft-versus-host disease: A condition in which the lymphocytes from a donor's stem cells recognize certain antigens on the recipient (patient) as foreign.

Graft-versus-leukemia effect: Occurs when the donor's lymphocytes attack the patient's leukemia cells directly and help in the eradication of the leukemia.

Granulocyte colony-stimulating factor: Growth factors given to activate production of cells.

Healthcare proxy: Document that limits the decision-making power to only those decisions about your medical treatment.

Hematopoietic growth factors: Drugs that increase blood cell counts.

Hemoglobin: The protein carried by red blood cells that delivers oxygen to the bodies tissues.

Hematologic remission: Remission defined by the blood counts' return to normal.

Hematologist: A specialist who sees and treats patients with malignancies (and other diseases) of the blood.

Hematopoietic stem cell: Referring to its ability to make all the cellular elements of the blood.

Hematopoietic stem cell transplantation: The process by which new stem cells are introduced into a patient.

HLA: See human leukocyte antigen.

HLA-matched sibling: Compatible sister or brother who is determined by testing to be matched at specific loci.

Human leukocyte antigen (HLA): The protein on the surface of all cells that must be matched for bone marrow transplants.

Hyperpigmentation: Darkened patches of skin.

Immune system: Complex system by which the body protects itself from outside invaders that are harmful to it.

Immunophenotyping: A laboratory test whereby these area's antigens can be measured on the surface of the leukemia cell.

Immunotherapy: Treatment that stimulates the body's own defense mechanisms to combat diseases such as cancer.

Immunosuppression: Condition of having a lowered resistance to disease. May be a temporary result of lowered white blood cells from chemotherapy administration.

Immunosuppressive therapy: Therapy to decrease the response of the immune system.

Incidence: The rate at which a certain event occurs, e.g., the number of new cases of a specific disease occurring during a certain period.

Induction chemotherapy: The initial phase of tratment using medications.

Informed Consent: Process of explanation to the patient of all risks and complications of a procedure or treatment before it is done. Most informed consents are written and signed by the patient or a legal representative

Intensification chemotherapy: Use of additional cancer drugs after remission to eliminate any remaining cancer cells.

Intravenously: Entering the body through a vein.

Leukemia: A malignancy of a white blood cell in which there is an abnormal accumulation of white blood cells in the blood and the bone marrow.

Leukocyte: A white blood cell or corpuscle.

Living will: Document outlining what care you want in the event that you become unable to communicate due to coma or heavy sedation.

Lymphocytes: Weakly mobile cells made in lymphoid tissue that are typical cellular elements of lymph and include cellular mediators of immunity; constitute 20%–30% of leukocytes of normal human blood.

Macrophage: A cell derived from a monocyte that functions to protect against infection and noxious substances.

Malaise: A condition marked by fatigue and overall poor feeling.

Metastasis: The spread of cancer from one part of the body to another through the lymphatic system or the bloodstream.

Microorganism: An organism of minute, microscopic size.

Molecular remission: Remission defined by analysis of small numbers of cells that indicate that a disease is totally eradicated.

Molecule: The smallest particle of a substance that retains the properties of the substance; composed of 1 or more atoms.

Monoclonal antibody: Antibody that specifically binds to a particular molecule on the surface of a certain type of leukemia or other cancer.

Monocyte: A type of white blood cell that is transported to tissues, where it turns into a macrophage.

Mucositis: A temporary but painful condition in which the lining of the inside of the mouth breaks down, making eating and swallowing difficult.

Myelodysplastic syndrome: A disease of the bone marrow stem cells in which the normal maturation of blood cells is altered.

National Marrow Donor Program: A large registry with millions of potential donors in its files for future stem cell transplants.

NMDP: See National Marrow Donor Program.

Neutropenia: A condition in which the body is depleted of important disease-fighting white blood cells.

Neutropenic diet: A diet that avoids foods that might carry harmful bacteria, such as raw meats or fresh fruits and vegetables.

Neutrophil: The most common granulocyte, a type of white blood cell.

Ommaya reservoir: A device inserted into the brain for the removal of fluid or instillation of medication.

Oncologist: A physician who specializes in cancer treatment.

Oncology: The science dealing with the physical, chemical and biologic properties and features of cancer, including causes, the disease process, and therapies.

Orally: Taken by mouth.

Palliative treatment: Therapy that relieves symptoms but does not alter the development of the disease. Its primary purpose is to improve the quality of life.

Pathogenesis: The origin and development of a disease.

Patient advocate: An individual who serves the needs of the patient, who may be empowered to act on his or her behalf.

Petechiae: Small red dots on the skin as a result of a very low platelet count.

Pharmaceuticals: Medications that are continuously being developed for future patient care.

Philadelphia-chromosome: The abnormal chromosome found in patients with CML.

Platelet: A cell formed by the bone marrow and circulating in the blood that is necessary for blood clotting.

Platelet transfusions: Procedures used in cancer patients to prevent or control bleeding when the number of platelets have decreased.

Port-a-cath: A device surgically implanted under the skin, usually on the chest, that enters a large blood vessel and is used to deliver medication, chemotherapy, and blood products; also is used to obtain blood samples.

Prevalence: The number of people alive with a particular disease at any moment.

Prognosis: A prediction of the course of the disease; the future prospect for the patient.

Prognostic factors: Factors that help to determine the severity of a disease.

Prophylactic treatment: Treatment geared to prevent disease or infection.

Protocol: A schedule of selected drugs and treatment time intervals known to be effective against a certain cancer.

Radiation oncologist: A specialist trained in the use of high-energy x-rays to treat cancer.

Radiation therapy: treatment with high-energy x-rays to destroy cancer cells.

Relapse: The reappearance of cancer after a disease-free period.

Red blood cells: Hemoglobin-containing cells that carry oxygen to the tissues.

Remission: Complete or partial disappearance of the signs and symptoms of disease in response to treatment; the period during which a disease is under control.

Risk factors: Anything that increases an individual's chance of getting a disease such as cancer.

Secondary cancers: A second site where cancer is found.

Secondary leukemia: A malignancy somewhat more common in patients previously treated with certain types of chemotherapy.

Side effects: Usually describes situations that occur after treatments. For example, hair loss may be a side effect of chemotherapy; fatigue may be a side effect of radiation therapy.

Staging: Evaluating the extent of the disease.

Standard protocol: Treatment generally recognized by the medical community as the standard of care.

Stem cells: A primitive type of cell from which all cells of a given organ or tissue arise.

Stem cell transplant: The process by which new stem cells are infused into a patient.

Subcutaneously: Injected under the skin.

Supportive treatment: Treatment with the goal of preserving the strength of the patient.

TBI: See total body irradiation.

T lymphocytes: Lymphocytes that directly attach themselves to virally infected or transformed cells to mediate their destruction.

Tissue: A collection of similar cells. There are four basic types of tissues in the body: epithelial, connective, muscle, and nerve.

Total body irradiation: Treatment in which the entire body is exposed to the same intensity of radiation, which is precisely determined by the radiation oncologist to remove all indication of disease.

Translocation: The movement of one piece of chromosome to another chromosome.

Trisomy 12: An extra chromosome 12 that is frequently present in patients with CLL.

Tumor: An abnormal tissue, swelling, or mass; may be either benign or malignant.

Veno-occlusive disease: A sometimes fatal condition that can lead to liver failure; requires rapid medical intervention.

WBC: White blood cells; a blood cell that does not contain hemoglobin; also called leukocyte.

Index

Index